Higher

Vibrational

Health

How to Shift Your Vibrations

for Self-Healing and Optimal Health

by

Tanya Jopson

www.guidancefromspirit.com

For general information about our products and services please contact our Customer Care Dept. of Guidance from Spirit within the United States of America @ (941) 822-4278.

Library of Congress Cataloging in Publication Data

Tanya Jopson 2014

Higher Vibrational Health: How to Shift Your Vibrations for Self-Healing and Optimal Health

ISBN 978-1475026306   1475026307

Health and Fitness

Printed in the United States of America

Dedication

*Appreciation of humanity and the collective gains we make
and continue to make as this incredible journey of wonder,
discovery and return to our highest vibration possible, unfolds*

and to

*Tyson and Ashley, who are shining examples of health, vitality,
and youthful exuberance while living life by honoring
their highest values.*

Contents

Introduction

A healthy disposition in life is often determined by what is seen in the physical environment of someone's existence. Are we able to, function, live and work at a sustained pace with minimal visits to the doctor or a low amount of bouts of illness? Do we exercise and take in adequate nutrition so we stay healthy? Are our thoughts inspiring and beneficial toward not only our own accountability for health, but also for enriching humanity? All of these questions are relevant when we set out to claim our life as healthy and not one of dis-ease.

But over the last ten years or so, the determining factor as to the degree of a person's health has shifted to include a deeper level of existence. A level that is not so easily seen, this level is the subtle Energy Body of an individual. The subtle energy level of existence includes the energy flowing through the Chakra centers and those energetic layers that go beyond the veil, between our physical existence and higher-self in spiritual existence.

It is these levels that I present in this book as I show how the pathways of energy travel from the deeper aspect of who you are to the grosser level of your physical existence. The subtle Energy-Body is where the effects of ill-health and disease can lay unexpressed as a very real energy presence, even before they become visible in our physical form.

Reaching these deeper levels of our whole self is not difficult when we are shown how. And often just a small effort in energy clearing and energy integration can cause a huge shift in how we feel and interact with the world of our everyday life.

Today, traditional health fields with complementary and alternative health practices are blending so that in working together, the patient or health-conscious person can err on the side of prevention over cure. The prevention of disease includes self-care and the maintenance of our energy field at vibrational levels which do not include dis-ease. Often, an energy shift can reward in such a way that a person will not experience a particular situation again, simply because we have essentially broken the cycle of its repetition by creating an environment which becomes unsuitable for disease to manifest.

Today, we have access to an abundance of energy-effective modalities that benefit our goal of well-being; these benefits are not only isolated at an energetic level but, more importantly yet, ripple out to benefit the actual health of our physical presence.

In this book, you will discover many of those modalities and hear stories of energy healing that defy logical explanation. Your energy presence is powerful and it is also a continuing aspect of you that finds its home in the creative source of reality itself. You can channel this creative essence from Source and send it forth into the world as your own unique expression. In order to channel this creative essence, your own energy field must be a clear pathway, uninhibited by what plays out in the human level of consciousness that causes blocks to receiving energetic impulses from our source of life. This book will highlight how energy blockages occur and what you can do to release them from the pathways of your energy field.

The quest for change in life is not always an easy undertaking. Change often conveys that all you presently believe to be a permanent reality, will now be revealed as not so. Often, it is this very revelation that we, as a human, resist. Because change for some people is a very frightening undertaking, and yet it is the only constant which moves us into a place of expansion, giving one a greater perceptional view of not only your own reality but the interconnected reality of humanity and its spiritual counterpart.

Intelligent creative energy flows throughout the universe, giving birth to the deeper beauty in all that is manifest. Moving within this energy, that creates harmonious, love filled life is a gift of free-will choice. Humans have free will to use this creative energy for manifestation of both a denser or lighter vibrational life. And so the potential for duality exists as we unconsciously or consciously make choices. Yes, you use that intelligent creative energy everyday in any way YOU choose.

Duality occurs when we believe that we are separate from the intelligent energy of the Creator.

Your higher-self as an energetic substance is closer in reflective content to the intelligent creative activity of the Creator's energy. And yet because of free-will you can choose to live mainly in the external world experiences and daily situations of a reality your biological eyes see.

You have for a moment traveled away from the higher consciousness of you, expanding into that which is a dense material reality, and often collectively low in vibrational content.

Your higher-self knows it is the reflective energy formation of the Creators essence, its goal is, to manifest the heaven we know deep within, that beautiful harmonious world we all vision.

Your higher-self waits patiently till you consciously choose to connect and call it forth. Therefore unifying the levels of your physical and higher-self into an integrated flowing vessel for higher conscious quality energy. In the process of embodying your higher-self energy you unify with the Creators essence. Your higher-self, is the storehouse for intelligent creative energy flow into the world.

Energy vibrations which are consciously called forth from our own higher-self are the reflective content of the intelligent creative energy vibrations of the Creator.

Connecting to and calling forth the Creator's energy from our higher-self, manifests in our world, content, experiences and lifestyles of an aligned vibration.

It is now time we honor our God-self and allow the loving intent of an intelligent creative Creator to produce through us an external world, that will mirror back all that we recognize as being of a higher vibration.

Within this book, we look at the human Energy-Body with the intent to clear any blockages of a mental, emotional or physical nature, thus allowing us to embody more of the spiritual energy essence, which is the healthy creative force of who we collectively are.

Chapter 1

Your Energy Presence

Welcome to *Higher Vibrational Health.* I hope you find the energy of my intent to write this book aligned with the energy of your attraction to the book itself. I was not always as fine-tuned toward the subject of energy and vibration as I am now. And I certainly did not hear about the human Energy-Body until about fifteen years ago. It was then that a huge "A-ha!" moment happened for me and life took a turn that I truly desired.

As I look back now, I see that my whole life was slowly building upon itself so that today, as I present the subject of energy and vibration, I am actually helping others to understand and use this information in a way that is beneficial to them. I am not going to even pretend for one moment that I knew in my early life that I would be involved in the subject of energy and vibration, because I simply did not. But I did have an early life inclination and tremendous desire to become a writer, something that I absolutely love to do. I was also extremely interested in spirituality and the interconnectedness of humanity at a deeper level. It is my current understanding that because of these interests along with my persistence and practice of healthy spiritual modalities that the knowledge about the nature of energy and vibration grew in my awareness so that it has now become my life work.

Further in this book, I present an in-depth look at the various forms of energy healing that are available today, but first, I feel it will serve you, the reader, if I present the Energy-Body layers so that you can grasp a clearer perspective of your own energy field as it relates to a larger spiritual presence. I will also show where and how energy blocks occur within your energy field and how energy healing shifts those blocks within our energetic presence, so that you can channel the clearer energy of creative Source into your everyday life.

So, let's visit the moment of your birth. You were born as a biological human who has a Source of Life fueling your physical presence that even today remains as a phenomenon. We all have an inner essence of life Source that keeps the biological doing what the biological is supposed to do. We often do not even think about this; we go about our day absolutely reliant that our Source of Life will be there within every moment that we need it. This Source of Life is intangible and we do not see its presence; we may ponder, wonder and investigate a bit, but generally our attention is on the external world, along with the responsibilities and experiences in which we find ourselves.

It is often not until our biological has some form of disruption or dis-ease that we may delve deeper in an effort to find why our biological presence has gone out of balance.

When we have certain physical ailments, or a presence of dis-ease, it is now known that they often originate from an energetic imbalance, and, if this is corrected, the ailment or dis-ease will likewise be corrected, as well.

So, what is this energy presence that has such a profound effect on our level of health? The presence is known as our Energy-Body, or field, and is shown in the following:

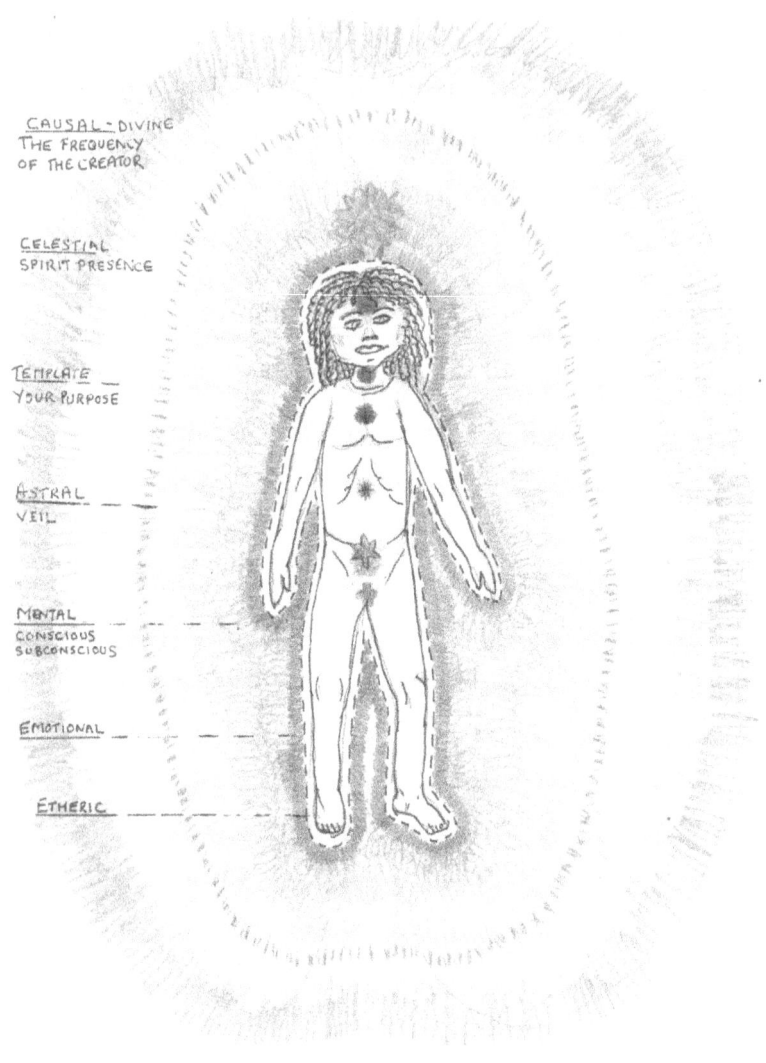

CAUSAL - DIVINE
THE FREQUENCY
OF THE CREATOR

CELESTIAL
SPIRIT PRESENCE

TEMPLATE
YOUR PURPOSE

ASTRAL
VEIL

MENTAL
CONSCIOUS
SUBCONSCIOUS

EMOTIONAL

ETHERIC

Think of your Energy-Body presence as a rainbow circled
around and within you, with each of the colors
functioning as specific type of energy for your physical

self. The layers are physical, etheric, emotional, mental and causal/spiritual.

All of the layers consist of electromagnetic energy, and even the physical layer is formed from this energy. The various layers of energy vibrate at a particular frequency, which are interconnected with levels of consciousness:

"Dr. David Hawkins has, arbitrarily, set a logarithmic scale of consciousness or the "map of consciousness." The levels accurately show where the person is on their path.... Just that you get a little taste of what is what: feeling shame and misery is under 50, infatuation/physical attraction is 145, pride is 150, courage is 200, and unconditional love is 525. Current global average vibration is around 207, though 98% of all people are under 200. The difference comes from the relatively few people who have a vibration way above average."

(http://getunstuck.university1000.com/self-improvement/what-is-your-vibrational-frequency)

When we understand, and embrace, that we are more than just a physical body, and that it is the energy/spirit body that manifests the physical body, we can now infer that anything that affects us energetically or spiritually will show up in the physical body and ultimately within our physical world.

The more transparent, or light-like, our layers are, the higher the vibrational frequency of our own signal.

The denser the layers are, the lower our vibrational frequency. This is usually caused by blocks, or stagnant energy that we can learn to process and transmute, which simply means we change, or move out, non-serving, or low, dense energy.

Let's look closer at:

The Subtle Layers of the Human Energy-Body

We are comprised of an Energy-Body of subtle layers. Any blocks or distortions in these vibrational layers will eventually make it to the physical self, and show up as some form of disease, or, if you prefer, "dis-ease."

Understanding how the layers of the Human Energy-Body function together is necessary to reverse and clear lower energy effects. It is also helpful for us to see that with deliberate intention we can actually consciously make changes to our energy field which then has an effect on our external reality. The following is an outline of the Human Energy-Body layering:

The Physical Energy-Body

Our physical body is a biological representation of the total frequency emission of our energetic self. This is the part of ourselves that uses our five senses when navigating the experiences and situations that are manifest within our reality.

All energetic content, whether imprinted from childhood, flowing in from higher-self as Spirit Guidance, or taken in from our external world will affect the physical body.

The Etheric (Astral) Energy Body

This layer of our Energy-Body is the blueprint for the physical body, and exists prior to it. It is the first layer of the Human Energy-Body that we do not see with physical sight unless we train ourselves to do so. As we look at the outline of our hand, we can pick up a subtle transparent hue, or outline of the hand itself; this area is evidence of the etheric energy.

The etheric contains the energy meridians, matrix and Chakra points that energy travels through to enter the physical world. In order for the spirit essence to form the physical, it moves through the energetic presence of the etheric, thus transforming into the lower etheric energy that is inherent within form itself.

Etheric utilizes life Source energy and impulses physical reality to sustain the energetic frequency necessary to maintain physical form in the configuration in which it is found now.

Any change that occurs in our etheric vibration alters the form previously created; the mental and emotional bodies precede the etheric and, therefore, have an effect upon it.

Every time that we think, we set in motion the mental energy within us, which then travels as a vibration to the etheric body.

When the etheric body sustains the vibrations of that thought by adding matching emotional vibrations, then that which is thought about will become manifest, due to the fact that the etheric energy sends that vibration further into the world we know as our everyday life.

While the etheric is important to inducing formation of our physical world, it is not the sole player in this co-create reality game.

The Emotional Energy Body

This subtle energy contains our emotional patterns, feelings and vibrations that display how we interact or react with other people and situations.

Emotions that are unexpressed, stay within the emotional energy field and cause havoc until they are processed and released; emotions exist and interpenetrate all the layers of the Human Energy-Body.

You can have a powerful thought, but, unless it is connected to an aligned emotional vibration, it will simply be incoherent for manifestation. We can all feel a stark difference in the way our body feels when we experience hatred or anger, and then love or peace; the difference between these feelings is the vibrational frequency that each holds.

Should we suddenly experience an unexplainable emotion, it could derive from the transference of an energy vibration emanating from someone who is in close proximity to us, or from the dislodging of a previously suppressed emotional blockage.

The Mental Energy Body

The mental energy field includes the gathering of our thoughts; it reflects our ability to string together cohesive lines of thought and it is where we construct images and ideas.

Our thoughts are powerful, since they have ability to create or destroy, and we would be wise to consider what we think about while we are thinking it.

The mental body is not limited to containing our own thoughts, but, as with the emotional body, when a sudden feeling occurs, the mental body is also capable of receiving the transference of a thought from another person's mental field and from the field of collective consciousness.

Often, the thoughts that fall into our subconscious mind are those that have been repeated often enough so that they become an accepted part of the subconscious in such a way that they create a permanent energetic pattern that can consistently affect our everyday life.

The Spiritual (Causal) Energy Body

This is our higher self, or I AM, presence and holds our master plan for this lifetime.

Few people spend enough time within the strata of their Energy-Body to harmonize with this layer, and yet it is from this area that we are so richly rewarded, as this is the layer which enables direct contact with our Source of Life.

As we learn to clear the Energy-Body layers that vibrate closer to the physical body through expansion of self-awareness and the cleansing of dense vibrations, we come to connect more and more with the energy of this particular layer of our self.

These collective energy layers make up the Human Energy Field, and they encompass and resonate vibrationally with each other. They are then, in turn, connected to the universal energy field by being encompassed within it.

The universal energy field is the life Source energy of the Creator. Everything is made from energy; the only thing that distinguishes one physical formation from another is the frequency of the energy at which it vibrates. The

Human Energy-Bodies are known as subtle energy because they are difficult to perceive with the five senses, but they are, indeed, very real and perceived through the practice of expanding awareness and tuning in to them.

Just as you personally have a Human Energy-Body, so, too, do all members of the human race. Our Energy-Bodies carry on communication with each other constantly, whether we feel it, know it, agree or disagree with it.

We are the resulting physical formation of originally unformed spirit energy, which is directly emanated from the source of all life. We in turn alter that energy formation with our own Energy-Body vibrations.

We connect with, and then flow, that life source energy toward our everyday life. With an authentic full embodiment of the spiritual layer of our Energy-Body, we come to feel and see our external reality from a balanced, cleared perception that contains the highest vibrational patterns.

What does this mean? It means we are empowered to connect with, communicate with, and become one with the original core content of the spirit-life source out of which, we are formed.

We then know our self, intuitively, as part of a unified existence and as one who is an expression of the Creator within our own reality; we are able to connect with all other Energy-Bodies at a non-physical, intangible point of reality.

Our energetic connection is that mode of communication that holds the least resistance, or burden of content, from our mental and emotional baggage. It is easy to communicate energetically to each other simply by bringing ourselves to an awareness, and acceptance, of this intention before it occurs.

Our being able to bring spiritual energy into our physical lifestyle requires that the layers of our mental and emotional bodies go through a renewing or clearing of denser states. These denser states are due to our desire to promote our own good to the world over that which seeks expression as guidance from spirit. Once the difference is understood we surrender to doing the work of Divine mind and this creates the momentum needed to raise our Human Energy-Body to higher and higher frequencies, thus giving our reality extended states of joy, harmony, love and enduring unity.

Chapter 2

How Energy Blocks Occur

Along with our energy field, we also have an energy matrix made up of meridian, or flow, lines of energy. These meridians act as channels for energy to travel through specific organs and systems. These are the energy pathways for the physical body and, being interconnected, are susceptible to blocks. The meridians travel from the area of the skin to deep within the muscles and organs. Traditional Chinese medicine works on these meridians with the use of acupuncture.

As a young child, we played and participated in life as a free spirit, learning and growing under influence from the people around us and the environment that surrounded us. If, as a child, we felt safe and loved, then we grew to see the world as a safe and loving place this also facilitated a clear sense of spirit flow from deep within .

If we were, on the-other-hand, humiliated and violated, then we grew to see the world as serving up more of these types of situations. The vibration of these denser modes of experience facilitated a closed off and more rigid type of existence in which we felt isolated and alone.

These different views of life shaped our perception of reality, but what we hold within our perception is not always of such an obvious nature to us. Our perception is formed because of the totality of experiences that we have and is in a constant changing flux. Renew a friendship and your perception changes. Experience a loss and your perception changes. Finish a college course and your perception changes.

Every experience alters our perception and either allows us to feel that life is beautiful, harmonious and worth our investment, or that life is dreadful and tough, causing us to want to withdraw.

Because, as a child, our energy field was also being affected at a deeper level, this also caused us to engage in a particular perceptional view. This perceptional view and the resonance effect of close-to-us energy caused our energy field to develop a set-point energy vibration. A set-point vibration occurs when a particular energy vibration becomes the normal range for a particular energy field, much the same as when two tuning forks become synchronized even when only one of them is activated. But since they are at close proximity to each other, both will soon harmonize because of the action of resonance, leading them to move at the same vibration.

When, as a child, we do not feel that we are in an environment that accepts who we are and how we want to express, we tend to shut down and withhold our expression. This lack of expression becomes an inner block within our energy field and that block continually sits there, waiting for expression. We then pick up the dominant energy vibration of that particular environment and our Energy-Body harmonizes with this vibration whether we like it or not.

It is my belief that most energy blocks come from the type of thoughts we have and these cause us to withhold expressing our emotions. Buried emotions form a block that can quite literally stay with us from our childhood into our adult years.

Our most impressionable times are those that cause a jolt to whom we thought we were, within what we thought the world was. This is shown as being in an experience that is incoherent with whom we are. When that occurs, we become out of sync and our vibration is altered to one that we do not resonate with in an adaptive way. So, it is not whether any environment or situation can be considered better than the one we presently have but whether we are compatible with the vibration we are encountering, and, if not, how are we affected as we assimilate to that vibration.

Some people have an innate ability to adjust and fit within any vibrational environment whereas others are deeply disturbed when they come across energy vibrations too far off from their normal signature vibration. In knowing about these energy and vibrations, you have the power to alter any future visions that you may have, and you can also erase past negative imprints.

That being said, if a child grew up in an environment loaded with violent behavior and humiliation; an environment of love would then be considered out of alignment with the energy vibration that had become that child's set-point reality. In such a situation, the environment filled with love would take a little time for someone to assimilate with, in order for it to then become the dominant vibration of a person raised in a violent household and who is, therefore, imprinted with violent levels of vibration.

So, energy blocks occur within our energy field when we internalize our feelings and do not express our emotions to others. They also occur when we do not express our ideas or thoughts because we do not feel confident enough to do so or have suffered ridicule because we have shared a particular thought before.

But energy blocks can also occur when we continue to behave in a way that we do not feel aligned to. This type of block occurs because we create a habit of action based on fear of change. Do you know someone who continues to attend and go through the motion of a particular type of work when they really want to do something totally different? This energy block is caused by the repetitive nature of continuous performance in an activity in which the person has little love or passion for doing. Frustration becomes the norm and complaining is a continuous output.

Another type of energy block occurs with regard to our relationships with other people. Do we find that we continually manifest and take part in relationships doomed to failure because we cannot move past a certain level of closeness with other people? We have no trust that getting close to someone will be a positive experience and, therefore, we subconsciously sabotage nearly if not all the relationships that we have.

An abundance energy block occurs when we view life as not able to give all that we want in any given moment. Often this is an imprinted belief taken on when someone has grown up in a working class family, of which the majority of people have done. This type of block is also strengthened when someone mistakes the saying, that money is the root of all evil and, therefore, not wanting to err on the side of evil they subconsciously repel money when it enters their environment. This type of energy block will reinforce the environment that you support in a low-level of vibration to show as real, any beliefs that you have about living in an abundant fashion.

If we do not believe that all needs are distributed from the Source of Creation and we strive to hold on to what possessions we have, because we fear a state of lack, we actually block our-self from receiving in an abundant way: we receive as we have sown and as our needs arise.

A creative energy block occurs when the frustrations of life hold your dominant attention. This means that in place of using spirit-energy to guide achievement, you are continuously placing your energy on the dramas of life and giving those dramas the focus of your energy and your creative power. We can always make a mountain out of a molehill when we fuel the molehill with the energy we could be using for a creative endeavor. Too many dramas in life cause an overwhelming feeling of helplessness; you have too many avenues in which you have placed your attention and, therefore, the strength of your energy is diluted into only fueling drama, and not being utilized for manifesting the creative ability that same energy could be used for.

Communication energy blocks occur when people of differing perceptions and beliefs simply do not hear the other person or accept, what they say without judgment. It is difficult to accept another point of view, of which there are as many as there are people, when we consider that only our own view is correct. I once engaged in conversation, with a person who because of their response taught me that while we live in the same world we can actually live in different realities. The person was going through a break up and I was trying to offer some words of wisdom, thinking I was getting through, the person turned to me and said, 'I don't have it within me to understand what you are saying." It hit me like a ton of bricks that I was talking as if he understood all that I did from my perception of reality. So I quickly adjusted what I was saying so that he could understand me.

It is also difficult, as a parent, to distinguish between our parenting role and the role as advocate for our child's independence. Each role requires a different form of behavior and when the two are not distinguished, perceived and acted upon in the right circumstances, we can find ourselves creating an energy block causing tension in the parent-child relationship.

Energy blocks also occur when we overly emphasis a particular action or habit. When we are not balanced in our participation in something and tend toward addictive behaviors and obsessions. This occurs when areas of life that should receive an equal share of our Life Source energy become neglected and slowly diminish due to a lack of energy to support its presence. This is witnessed in someone who favors alcohol or drugs; at the onset they channel energy into all areas of life, but, over time, the addictive behavior gains the majority of energy and the other areas of life, such as relationships, career, fun, hobbies, spiritual pursuits and finances all eventually have less and less energy and, therefore, less and less presence in the forefront of an addictive person's life.

The lack of adequate or optimal nutrition is also a way in which an energy block occurs, especially with regard to the consumption of genetically modified food, about which we dedicate a chapter later.

Many blocks occur with regard to our Chakra system which are the gateways of energetic flow into the reality that we live. The Chakras also draw energy into our energy field from places and environments in which we find ourselves. Our Chakras are connected to various biological systems and their energetic flow determines our optimal health. Here, we take a closer look at the Chakras, what occurs if they are blocked, operating at an optimal vibration, and the food that enhances their energetic flow.

Chakra	Conditions if Blocked	Optimal Vibration	Enhanced by Food
Root: base of spine; color: red	Lack of autonomy; dependency on others; eating disorders,	Grounded; secure; healthy; fit; easy ability to manifest material goals	Protein, root vegetables and red tomatoes, strawberries, cranberries, etc.
Sacral Chakra: lower abdomen; color: orange	Lack of passion in life, overly attached to possessions, smother and engulf people	Healthy boundaries; easy to give and receive love; share creative abilities	Fats and oils; smoked salmon; carrots, curry, apricots, pumpkins and mango
Solar Plexus; stomach; color: yellow	Fear of rejection; little will power; power struggles; control issues; repressing anger; tendency to lie	Self-respect; self-discipline; self-confidence; ability to take action to manifest desires	Complex carbohydrates, corn, ginger, bananas, yellow lentils, oats, rice and rye
Heart Chakra: heart; color: green	Inability to empathize or forgive mistakes; possessiveness for love; need others to complete them	Kind, generous, welcoming and open; tranquility and acceptance;	Chlorophyll and green asparagus, avocado, kale, green grapes, micro-greens and sprouts

		shows love regardless of past experiences	
Throat Chakra: neck area; color: blue	Inability to speak clearly; a creative block; only say what we think others want to hear	Express honestly; nurture a talent such as writing or singing; calibrates our frequency and attracts matching experiences	Sea plants, soups, sauces, juices and fruits
Third Eye Chakra: pituitary, hypothalamus and pineal gland; color: indigo	Headaches, sinus issues, depression and anxiety; difficulty in remaining focused or focused too intently on one thing	Receive wisdom from our inner world; free of attachment to a situation, a belief, an outcome, a person, etc.; clear	Blackberries, blueberries, purple grapes, wine, red onions, purple potatoes

		perception	
Crown Chakra: just above the top of the head; the pure essence that connects to All; color: violet or white	Believes in own abilities and lacks faith in Divine Consciousness as the lead for reality	Ability to be fully connected spiritually while able to be grounded to physical existence	Plum, eggplant but mainly receives sustenance from air, sun and love

Put together with information from www.chakrashack.com,

Clearing our own energy field from dense energy and aligning to the flow of Higher Vibrations from Source is a form of energy healing.

So too is understanding that we are not alone in the journey we take here on earth. We are accompanied by, our higher-self that spiritual aspect of who we are that does not interfere in our growth but assists us when called upon. While we may have garnered a few energy blocks from the lifestyle, thinking and suppression of our emotions these blocks are actually vehicles through which we learn to embody the energy of our higher-self in our everyday life.

Chapter 3

How Energetic Imbalance Becomes Disease in the Body

Is healthcare keeping you sick? I recently came across healthcare information that seemed to operate at a reverse to how western healthcare operates and I must say I actually love the concept. It comes from Chinese medicine: *historically, a Chinese doctor was paid a retainer to keep his patients healthy; if a patient became sick, the doctor would not be paid until the patient's health returned and in some cases the doctor had to refund the retainer.*

The five arms of Chinese medicine are:

1. *Acupuncture;*
2. *Herbal medicine;*
3. *Massage and bone setting;*

43

4. *Martial and meditative arts, and,*

5. *Dietary therapy.*

www.seqclinic.com

The Chinese have traditionally worked on the energy systems of the human presence with a goal of maintaining health and avoiding the occurrence of disease.

With the increase today of energy healers in the west and the growth of vibrational medicine, I feel we, too, are moving toward the prevention of dis-ease through the maintenance and balance of our energy fields.

We are still in the infant stages of this development but we can each take part and work on our own energy systems to ensure health and not fall victim to dis-ease. Once disease is noted in us, it now has our personal energy through attention we place on it, and it is often difficult to remove our attention when it is directed toward the existence of something by a few people.

How does disease manifest from our energetic presence? We saw earlier that the energy field is the building block of our physical vessel, and that every experience and situation has an effect on the vibrations of our energy field. This occurs because of the in-and-out flow of energy through the Chakra gateways. Often, a blockage, or incoherence, occurs between fields of energy, and these cause a disruption in vibration or a block in energy flow.

When a block occurs as a result of suppressing energy, then the flow of Life Source from the more spiritual to the grosser aspect of self is slowed, meaning that that particular part of us along the pathway of the meridian is now not receiving the level of Life Source energy needed for optimum maintenance. Over time and with a lack of vital Life Source energy, the body part correlating to the system affected by the block begins to show physical symptoms of this limited energy flow.

We define health as the tangible results in our physical existence being in harmony with our own inner energy flow of optimum Life Source Energy. This means we have an Energy-Body, or Spiritual Essence, which allows the highest form of energy to flow through us and out into the world. When we are in the flow, so to speak, the effects can be:

- Clear thinking and heightened concentration;
- A relaxed state even during chaos;

- Vitality and increased energy;

- Increased intuition and awareness;

- Recognition of synchronistic events;

- A feeling of unity and connectedness with others;

- Ability to easily find solutions, and,

- Appearance of creative ideas and visions to achieve.

We are not the ultimate Creator of ourselves and, therefore, we receive our life force from That which created us and created all things. This life force is the higher intelligent energy force that can run through our energy systems if the pathways are open to receive.

During the act of energy healing, or Reiki, the practitioner's hands are guided to the area of the body that has a degree of lesser Life Source Energy than the rest of the client's energy field. The energy exchange that occurs between the two then brings the area of lesser energy up in vibration; this is what causes a shift in the recipient's energy field.

In my early days of working with energy, I worked with crystals and channeled energy through my hands. I did not actually touch a person and found that my hands, if placed just a few inches away from a person's skin, would transfer energy so that the person would feel warmth. In fact, one time I asked my son to hold out his hand so I could show him how energy moves from one field to another and he quickly pulled his hand away, saying that his hand had become hot.

I never studied any particular healing modality but just felt that what I was doing was because of some inner guidance to do so. The following is a story which occurred about ten years ago:

I was living in Lakeland, Florida, with my husband and daughter. My husband at that time was in a stressful job, and he seemed too often to get bouts of kidney stones. The pain would relegate him to bed, and I would often think of the energy play that was causing the physical symptoms. I had just cleared my crystals by placing them in sea salt and leaving them outside the night before under the rays of a new moon. This was something I had just finished reading about.

Well, this particular day my husband had returned from a doctor's visit where an ultrasound had confirmed a kidney stone, and he was informed that it was of a size that he could pass. He went to bed in some discomfort and just wanted to sleep his way through the episode. As I went about my own business, the idea came for me to use my crystals and hands to remove the kidney stone. So, as he slept, I set to task; I quietly put the crystals around the edge of the bed using my crystal healing book as to where each particular crystal should be placed. Then, I knelt beside the bed facing his back and put my hands out and silently requested that the Creator remove the stones. As I directed my hands to where I thought the kidneys were located, I felt a power of energy pull my hands to another area close by. I shifted my hands slightly and it was then that the bottom crystal on the bed flew to the floor. It was a rose quartz. Now, I certainly know the difference between something falling and something being propelled, and this was definitely the latter. It was then that I felt an incredible wellspring of compassion for humanity, and I felt tears fall down my face because my inner desires to see humanity live in peace and health came to the surface of my existence. I knew that a more powerful energy had entered my space and so I surrendered to what was happening. I felt my hands guided into performing small circular motions and I requested, "Take this kidney stone far into the universe and smash it into a million pieces so it cannot hurt anyone again." It was then I heard, "Plant a seed." I thought, "I can do that," and then heard, "Not you, Brit [my husband]."

I picked up my crystals, wrapped them and put them back in the glass container in which I keep them. I exited the room with Brit none-the-wiser for what had transpired while he slept. I went into the laundry room and looked at the mango seed that was drying on the window sill. I knew this was the seed to be planted, but wondered how I was going to convince Brit to plant it.

Shortly after, a friend of mine arrived from Sarasota on a visit for the day. I made some tea and we sat and chatted. I told her all about my experience with the crystals and the kidney stone. Just then, Brit walked out from the bedroom and said he felt better and felt no pain or discomfort whatsoever. So I explained how he didn't have a kidney stone anymore and that he should plant a seed and told him there was the one in the laundry room. He walked to the laundry room, picked up the seed, looked at it, and put it back on the sill. I knew by the way he put it down that he had no intention of doing anything with it, and within a short period of time, he was back in pain, back in bed, and then, within a few hours, in an ambulance on his way to the hospital. I was reeling as I knew there was no kidney stone; I said to my friend, "I don't know how he could have such pain when he doesn't have a kidney stone anymore." Neither of us could understand what had taken place, but I knew it was because he had not planted the seed.

My friend left to drive back to Sarasota and I was just gathering my stuff to head to the hospital when Brit showed up at the door. The Emergency Room had called his doctor, who had performed whatever procedure they do to remove a kidney stone. After the procedure, the doctor reported to Brit that he did not have to remove the stone as the pieces were too small; he said, "It looked as if the stone has been broken into a million pieces," and that he would just pass them.

The doctor's explanation of the stone breaking into a million pieces cemented to me what I knew all along. My request to the Universe to remove the stone was heard and I had received exactly as I had requested. This was a big lesson for me in the fact that when we make vibrational or energy healing requests, we must be careful of the way we actually word our request.

Later, as I walked down the hallway to bring Brit a cup of green tea, I overheard a small segment of a conversation he was having with someone on the phone. He said, "I can't explain it, but the doctor said it looked like it had broken in a million pieces."

At least, if nothing else, that episode expanded the awareness of all concerned, so that using and requesting the universe to make a physical change by aligning with a more powerful energy, was something about which we all can learn more.

While I had attempted at that time to work on a physical symptom that I knew my husband was having, there may have been telltale energetic signs that the kidney stone was forming, a possible pre-physical energy state that could be adjusted before any stone was able to manifest within the body. At that time, I knew little about the ability to clear an energy-field of the influence that would develop into a physical ailment. Today, we have advanced in this area and our understanding and abilities are growing everyday.

What are some symptoms that arise from distortions in an energetic field? We all know the obvious such as the flip-flop of our stomach when we are feeling anxious; feeling anxious is a signal that our level of self-confidence is low. This correlates to our solar plexus, or our energy gateway related to our stomach.

What about consistent migraines? We know that the third eye Chakra is an energy gateway that, when in balance, cultivates more of a free-spirit person who goes with the flow and is not overly attached to outcomes in material existence. Migraines are a sign that our energy is being forcefully intentionalized toward an outcome that is heavily materialistic and inclined to and causing strain with the energy of the third eye Chakra.

Even though people on a spiritual path gain knowledge about what occurs of a mystical nature, we also have to bring energy from within our spiritual Chakras into the physical reality that we live.

What happens when an imbalance occurs while doing so? Let's look at a situation that occurred to me: Almost fifteen years ago, I divorced my first husband, moved into a small house and set out with determined intent to realize life of a spiritual nature, My food was completely vegetarian, I only drank water, and I meditated five to six hours every day, exercised with weights, and ran the beach three or four times a week. Apart from my job, I had lost touch with reality as I had known it. I had very little in the way of conversation with people and just lived in an isolated reality of my creation, fully believing that Gaia was expanding into a euphoric state and that all people were good. On the surface, this may not seem so bad, but I was way out of balance with what the rest of society was doing; no, I didn't seem concerned about that. The physical symptoms that manifested were an inability to make decisions about anything that was of a physical nature. I was so into the flow of being a divine being that I was not grounded enough to function in the everyday reality in which I had to live. I lost the ability to connect and communicate with my sons; I missed much in their growing up. So even at higher levels of spiritual practice, there is still the potential to have incoherence with what is going on around you, so much so that life goes on and you are not truly involved in it. I have forgiven myself for not being available for my sons and know that I would not be who I am today without that experience.

As mentioned at the end of the last chapter our experiences occur for our own evolution, guided by involvement of our higher-self. But what occurs when those experiences turn out as something we find distasteful. How are we supposed to handle the processing of this type of experience so that it does not become a block within our energy field?

All experiences aid our evolution even those that we complain about, dislike, find troubling or just downright hate. All experiences aid us in releasing traits such as criticism, slander, jealousy, judgmentalism, sarcasm, denigration, intolerance, violent impulses, hatred, anger, lying, cheating, stealing etc. When we accept that what occurs to us is not a prearranged situation but that it gives us the opportunity to act from a higher vibrational aspect we can see how each experience is an opportunity to express love in action.

We are not limited within any situation we have only been trained to believe that we are.

So how is a situation able to give us an empowered worldview? Each situation that we experience mirrors to us content that is still vibrationally operable within our own energy field. In order to function as our higher-self there will be certain elements of our physical nature that are not aligned with the divine nature of our-self. These elements or behaviors, thoughts, ideas are a construct of our human existence. When we see another person as a liar or a thief we have to look at the element within us that is manifesting this and ask, for what reason are we doing so. The world mirrors to us what we send out to it. While a person may steal from us, are we in-fact stealing from someone or something. Or do we hold judgment about those who steal. If so, then we will continue to experience this energetic occurrence until we alter our own vibration in regards to it.

Lets look at all that we believe is bad or dark. Firstly, we all have the potential to use energy in any of the ways in which energy is used. When we have participated in something that we judge ourselves for, we tend toward denial of its existence and create a secret space within to hide our indiscretions even from our self. This is known as our shadow and when we least expect it, our shadow will remind us of its presence. Often, what is known as, the dark-night-of-the-soul is our-self facing the shadow that we have buried. It is where all of our fears, addictions, wrongdoings, harmful ways, and less than favorable characteristics are faced in order for us to compassionately forgive our-self for burying them. When we realize that we are not free of creating shadow material, we are then able to shine light on the contents, so that we can truly embrace that our experience of these moments were necessary when we experienced them. It is often difficult to face our-self in the mirror knowing that we may have caused another harm, but even more so, loving our-self despite that experience.

Our human experience is not a journey that embodies only bliss. But totally denying that we have emotions and thoughts that we consider less than favorable will enable the shadow self to grow thereby blocking more of the divine light that seeks expression in our days.

Forgiveness is a process of revelation, acceptance and infusion of light and love on any situation that calls for healing before it becomes a vibration of dis-ease in our everyday life.

Can we collectively erase this element of dis-ease?

If we look at the big picture and ponder the path that humanity has taken regarding dis-ease, there are some promising signs to see. We have already wiped out some forms of disease from the collective reality that we all live; diseases such as polio, plague and smallpox were once prevalent and now only found in smaller isolated areas, if at all. How these diseases diminished or disappeared is not of paramount importance, but that they have shifted from dominance to rarity is a positive sign in regard to the diseases of today that have a more prevelant presence. When we look at the vibrational essence of civilization at the time that these diseases were prevalent, we can see a connection that the mind-of-man held certain characteristics that could be relational to manifestation of those diseases. Mankind held and emitted superstitious beliefs in witchcraft, ignorance of personal hygiene, and prevalence of subjugation of women, as well as low self-value and worth. Mankind truly lived in an energetic space of survival.

Shifting forward from those days to the nineteenth century, when the above diseases started to diminish what happened to the collective energy of humanity so that the manifestation of these diseases diminished? I believe that in those days, we did not consciously make a choice to eradicate particular diseases, but, somehow, somewhere in the collective subconscious of humanity, we did make that choice. And, so, we live to reap the rewards. One of those rewards was a great influx of spiritual information that would help humanity to overcome their survival instincts and reassess how the mind can have an affect in one's life. This, in turn, raised our collective energy vibration so much so that those types of diseases could no longer find a matching vibration for their presence to be sustained in our everyday collective reality.

Now we come to a collective provocation: If there is a correlation between our energy vibration and the state of health, not only individually but collectively, then just what is *it* that would facilitate our collective eradication of cancer, AIDS and other pandemics?

When we collectively learn and collectively act, we collectively gain. What about our collective use of the energy of intention, not only individually, but by creating a unified group force so that a Tipping Point of Transformation is reached which would raise our collective vibration high enough for cancer, AIDS and other prominent diseases to no longer have a matching vibration within the mass consciousness of humanity in order for them to become manifest.

In order for the collective subconscious of humanity to rise in vibrational frequency, we can each do our unique part. We can bring to our own awareness any shadow content that we have buried and forgive ourselves whole heartedly because our experiences within life and with each other, are product of universal laws aiding our souls growth and are a way for us to embody more of our divine higher-self energy whilst in human form.

The more we work with and understand the nature of our energy-spirit connection the easier it becomes to accept that we are on track with our evolution, while our evolution is assisted by learning about energy modalities and how they give to our overall health?

Chapter 4

An In-Depth Look at Various Forms of Energy Healing

Energy Healing is no longer isolated to some small, far out-of-the-way place with a village elder holding the title Shaman. But Energy Healing can now be found in any holistic spa and as a very real topic of discussion in government meetings and many research papers. When something increases in the popular culture so much that the government can no longer ignore its presence, it then becomes worthy of being investigated to the greatest extent possible.

But Energy Healing has taken place for thousands of years and will continue to do so. The following Energy Healing methods are all mentioned as areas of inquiry by the National Center for Complementary and Alternative Medicine, which is a government-based organization.

Complementary medicine works alongside conventional medicine, while alternative medicine is used in place of conventional medicine. The following is my own interpretation of these methods, because the government site often states, in regard to these modalities, "...not enough evidence that they are effective," which is understandable as the government only started looking at these modalities roughly ten years ago.

Acupuncture

Acupuncture is an ancient Chinese modality that is gaining in western use. I have never personally experienced acupuncture but a good friend of mine has; here is her story: One day, she was sitting at her job as a bookkeeper, and, over the course of the day, she had developed a severe headache. A colleague in the office who performed acupuncture, asked her what was the matter. She explained about the headache and her colleague said, "Wait there while I go and get my acupuncture needles and put them in your ears." My friend said, "The thought of having needles stuck in my ears was not such a welcoming thought," so she was thinking of ways to get out of it. Now, my friend admits she is a skeptic and just wanted to get home to lie down.

Her persuasive colleague, however, had her sit in a chair and proceeded to twist and tap the end of about four to six needles into each side of her head at the location of her ears. The acupuncturist said to her, "Just relax," and my friend said that as she did, she suddenly felt a rush of something from the back of her head, over the top, and toward the front. She said, "It felt like water," and when I asked her if she felt the energy, she said, "Why, yes, that was what it was and...the headache was immediately [and] completely gone."

I have also come across news that acupuncture is gaining in use as the anesthesia of choice by some doctors who do tonsillectomies on children. It is also being used as a measure to reduce pain after surgery.

Alexander Technique

I was introduced to this method of body awareness when a friend of mine, who is a yoga teacher, shared that she was practicing this methodology to enhance her yoga teaching abilities. I am still intrigued by the practice because I felt it related in a very clear way to the first step in my course, *Raise Your Vibration*. That first step is Expanding Awareness, and the Alexander Technique teaches by enlightening us to the movements of our own body. F. Matthias Alexander showed how we can think of ourselves as moving in a certain way, but with observation, we may find that we are not, in fact, using our body in the best way for optimum kinesthetic functioning. This, in turn, can add to the stress and anxiety of an already difficult life. The technique goes on to show various exercises and shifts in kinesthetic movement that alter the energy flow of our body. When we begin to pay attention to our posture and movements to assess their fluidity, we are essentially checking in on our presence in the world and living more in the moment. This is a level of awareness that few people achieve because their attention is directed more toward being entertained by whatever is in front of them.

Ayurveda

I studied Ayurveda many years ago at the Holistic Healers Academy. After checking with the National Council on Complementary and Alternative Medicine, I was surprised at the limited attributes that they quoted as being incorporated in this method of health care. They placed heavy emphasis on the fact that Ayurveda uses herbs for treatment, but made little reference to anything else. They also stated that too little was known to equate the practice as being effective. I wonder where they are getting their information because Ayurveda is actually over five thousand years old and is considered one of the oldest form of health treatments.

I was introduced to Ayurveda as the Science of Life and that this incorporated mind, body and soul balance. These are the areas I covered:

- Breathing exercises;
- Rubbing the skin with infused oils;
- Using mantras;
- Yoga;
- Weekly fasting to remove toxins from the body;
- Herbal medicines to balance *doshas*, and,
- Use of food to balance *doshas.*

As you can see, Ayurveda is not only limited to the use of herbs and really covers the mind, body and soul. I also learned that time frames within a day correlate with the energy cycles of the *doshas* (type of energy we have dominant within our energy field) and that performing certain tasks at certain times of the day are more beneficial than doing them at other times. For example, we would want to gear a task requiring mental agility to the time of day associated with *Vata* because it is during that time when you are most alert and creative.

The daily dosha clock runs as follows:

- 6:00 am – 10:00 am: *Kapha* - best time to awaken as the energy is conducive to a calm relaxed state;

- 10:00 am – 2:00 pm: *Pitta* - you are at your most active, and appetite is at its peak between 12:00 -1:00 pm;

- 2:00 pm – 6:00 pm: *Vata* - this is when you will feel most mentally alert and creative; dinner is best eaten before six because the next cycle is in the calm, relaxing energy state and not the best for digestion;

- 6:00 pm – 10:00 pm: *Kapha* - the perfect energy to unwind after a day's activities and maybe to perform yoga or meditation so the body and mind are at the vibration to go to sleep easily;

- 10:00 pm – 2:00 pm: *Pitta* - this active energy occurs while you sleep so the body is able to repair and renew cells, and,

- 2:00 pm – 6:00 am: *Vata* - during this phase, we actively process the content of the mind and, later, we either recall our dreams or don't, but they occur during this time.

The year is also divided into the *dosha* energy cycles and, with attention, you may notice that you can easily figure the cycles by the way you feel and behave during each time of the year.

Biofeedback

Biofeedback is the cornerstone of an expanding and wide range of equipment that essentially provides a client, with biological feedback about a physiological condition they may want to improve. The equipment measures biological responses and is a way to prove to a client how they are coping in response to certain stimuli. Biofeedback is used for physical, emotional and mental assessment, and records such changes in someone as muscle tightening, increase in heartbeat, sweat, temperature, etc.

An advance on the biofeedback technique, is the introduction of biopulser; this is a piece of equipment that goes even further by providing feedback at deeper levels of an individual's organs and energy field.

Crystal Healing

This topic seems to have as many people saying *nay* as it does people saying *yay*. The reason that people come out in such a powerful way against there being any benefit to crystal healing is because they honestly do not feel any sensation from the energy presence of crystals and they, therefore, cause their own block to crystals having a benefit, and so they live as they expect. I recall during the study of a Jose Silva course years ago, the quirky little statement that in order to manifest something you had to expect it, project it, and accept it. Unfortunately, some people mis-heard this and now they expect it, project it, and then reject it. For those people who reject crystal energy as being beneficial, it is because they have already turned off the possibility, and, therefore, they are no longer of a coherent energy to feel and accept it.

Crystal healing works by placing crystals on or around the body. The crystals draw out the negative content, such as energy blocks, and entrain their healing vibration to your energy field.

Curandero

Curandero translated means <u>healer</u>. They are frequently a tribal elder who restores the relationship between people, the earth, plants and animals. Curanderos use a range of modalities such as prayer, massage, herbal supplement and talk therapy. They work on the internal states of a person and do not accept that disease comes from germs, but that it arises from an imbalance in the mental and emotional states. They also attribute disease to evil spirits and curses.

Deep Breathing

Deep breathing, whether during meditation or simply as a practice, works to oxygenate the blood and cells of the body. Germs and disease do not thrive in an oxygenated host. Alongside this benefit, oxygen carries Life Source energy into every cell and acts to restore any low energy places. Recall that we said earlier that without Life Source energy, a particular part of the body will begin to atrophy and die.

Energy Healing

Energy Healing is any modality that works on the inner vibrational energy field to manifest change in the physical layer of a person's existence. These vibrational changes are often indicated by visible, physical symptoms but do not respond by treating the symptom as such, but, instead, by treating the underlying cause, which could be mental, emotional, and/or of a subconscious content that has occurred in a past life context still awaiting to be dealt with. Ascertaining whether someone has an energy block, is dealing with an energy vampire, or has negative energetic cords to untie, all help the Energy Healer in working with the client to re-balance the energy-field and teach that client how to support their own field in balance.

Espiritista

An Espiritista is someone who performs ritual and healing to exorcise evil spirit energy from a person's energy presence.

Feldenkrais

The Feldenkrais Method teaches awareness of habitual neuromuscular patterns and rigidities so that new ways of movement are explored with the goal of increasing sensitivity and efficiency. The method focuses on the intricate relationship between movement and thought, increased mental awareness and creativity accompany this movement. I am having a little chuckle here, maybe that is why office environments now offer walking stations with a computer attached, as the new office furniture!

Guided Imagery

Guided imagery is used to connect with the subconscious content of a client. When asked to close your eyes and allow an image to come to the forefront of your inner sight that image is often related or a clue to an issue that you may be experiencing. Often the person who is facilitating the process will then ask questions about the image and what it personally means to the client. Another way that guided imagery is used is to actually direct the client to forming an image based on verbal clues of a facilitator. This form of imagery can guide a client toward seeing themselves as a healthy human and reconnect them to the memories and subconscious content of a time that they remember before they showed symptoms that are unsettling. This is done to alleviate stress, depression, and any number of ailments that a client has in the forefront of their awareness. The premise is that what we focus on grows in our reality and therefore a healthier image constructed in the mind will become the main focus and therefore move to grow in our reality.

Hypnosis

I was introduced to Hypnosis by an outstanding hypnotist Alicia D. Cramer. My experience is that a hypnotist bypasses the sabotaging content of the conscious mind and connects with the subconscious wellspring of all that is empowering for your own life. I studied hypnotherapy as a way to broaden my understanding of the way in which content imprinted in our energy field and therefore also our consciousness, conditions our expression in life toward either success or failure. I am a big fan of hypnotherapy and especially of people like Alicia Cramer who teach you how to effectively use self-hypnosis to increase confidence and achieve your goals.

Massage

There is nothing like the therapeutic or healing touch of a good massage, whether it is a light soothing gentle Swedish massage or a deep tissue massage, used to get right into the inner layers of the muscles. The magic of touch is clear from the soothing massage of a parent to lull a baby to sleep to the caring touch of a caregiver when someone is sick. We have to stop looking only at what transpires during a physical action and more at the unseen phenomena when we engage in the world. There is far greater activity in the unseen aspect of our existence then we could ever see in the part of reality that our vision picks up on.

Touch matters and energy is transferred and stimulated during the process of massage. The benefits are numerous some being, the reduction of stress, and muscle tension, the regulation of digestion and general overall feeling of relaxation and wellness.

Massage can also be combined with essential oils so that the added benefit of aromatherapy is achieved.

Meditation

Meditation is a powerful gift that you can easily give to yourself. It is a modality used for eons and now has documented scientific benefits which are found at Pub Med gov website.

One of the most recent Harvard studies shows that meditation aids in curbing the mind from its incessant wandering and flitting from one thought to another. Researchers have discovered a connection between the state of a mind trained in meditation and the resulting state of happiness in that person. A person whose mind is in 'default mode network' or always on guard because the mind is left to wander has a less happy state.

People who meditate develop a mind state that is more clued into their presence in the moment and as it relates to the world as opposed to people who do not meditate who are more clued into the *me* thoughts which place their attention on their own worries and concerns in life.

Meditation is an enhancement to changing the wave patterns within the brain and this alters the wave patterns of the energetic field.

Progressive Relaxation

Progressive relaxation is a technique I have used. During my early days of meditation I found it difficult to switch off from my immediate surroundings and so would start at my feet by tensing the muscles and then slowly releasing the tension to totally relax them. I used this on each muscle group from my feet to my head and found that my body became totally relaxed after doing so.

Qi gong

In Chinese Qi means energy and Gong means cultivation. Qi pronounced *Chee*. Qi Gong teaches how to harness the energy that runs through your meridians and use that energy for self-healing. The energy that comes into the body is from a divine source and holds the code for the best possible version of our life. Embodying this energy changes the dynamics of our life so that life alters and reforms, becoming the best one that we vision. Health is part of that best life. So as we cultivate the use of our energy we can direct the Qi to self-heal any areas of our body that are not at their best formation.

Quantum Entrainment

This is not something I have experienced,

Quantum Entrainment quietly activates the autonomic nervous system to spontaneously and immediately create an atmosphere in which deep healing can take place. This amazing self-help method is easy to use and needs no previous knowledge, it can be applied by everyone! And what is most astonishing: Not only does the treated person receive deep, restful healing but the person who is using QE will also experience an immediate, prolonged sense of well-being." Dr. Frank Kinslow

Reiki

Reiki is an ancient form of hands-on-healing. History dates Reiki back to the Indian Nepal border in 620 BC. In the energy modality of Reiki a practitioner becomes the Reiki and acts as a channel as the spiritually guided life force energy flows through his vessel to mesh with another person's energy field. The higher frequency vibrations of the energy from spirit essence to physical presence will have a beneficial result on both the practitioner and the recipient. This modality is usually passed from Reiki Master to student by way of attunements and includes learning precepts (guidelines), techniques, hands-on healing, symbols and mantras, and a blessing called Reiju. Reiju asks that you receive whatever is needed in your life at this moment for your souls growth.

Shamanism

Shamanism is found across the world, and its practice spans many thousand years. Pre-dating all organized religions, it nonetheless has common threads of practice which unite shamans of all nationalities and all times, from the most distant past to the present day. There is some evidence to suggest that humans were practicing forms of shamanism as far back as the Palaeolithic, and certainly evidence for Mesolithic and Neolithic shamanism is widespread and in many indigenous cultures today it not only survives but is experiencing a resurgence. It is a primary and primal form of communicating with spirits and the spirit world, of understanding and interacting with the universe. By becoming a 'walker between the worlds' the shaman, acting as messengers and intermediaries between the mortal world and the realm of spirits can bring wholeness, protection, healing and knowledge direct from the spirit realm for use by all their community or tribe.

Http://www.danuforest.co.uk

<u>Sobador</u>

"The verb sobar means to knead, rub or massage. A sobador(male) or sobadora (female) is a person who, by massaging or kneading, treats sore muscles, sprains, tenseness and so on. They treat by massaging, rubbing, or kneading the affected part of our body. The sobadores do not have formal training, but they often follow a set procedure in the treatment

It is also important to note the cultural difference. The concept of a massage for the non-Hispanic is that it is many times for pleasure or relaxation. For the Hispanic, the massage (sobada) almost always is performed for healing purposes.

A sobador might well work only on the material level using his hands and perhaps an aromatic oil or a poultice or even a tea. But, a sobador might also heal even an ill that exists deep beneath the surface of the skin-indeed, perhaps in the nervous system or in the mind. That sobador might be said to operate on the psychic level as well. There are sobadores who have been said to cure paralysis

Most operate from their homes and, as always, the best advertisement is by word of mouth. More often than not, the session may involve confidences and advice from the sobador. One told me at one session that "what is said in this room, stays in this room." It also may involve a transmission of healing power from the hands to the affected body part. All healers believe that they have a special gift, called a don, from God to heal.

A sobada may also involve covering the forehead and sides of head with a heat-producing herb. Then the ears are covered by the healer's hands to produce more heat. A passage is produced so that negative feelings and "males" (negative thoughts) may pass from the inside of the body through the ears into the healer's hands.

The clientele of a good, reputable sobador will consist of Hispanic and non-Hispanic and even children. I have seen families bring their children, a non-Hispanic bring his son, and an entire family bring the grandmother to seek relief from her pains."

mexconnect.com

Tai chi

This gentle form of exercise can prevent or ease many ills of aging and could be the perfect activity for the rest of your life.

Tai chi is often described as "meditation in motion," but it might well be called "medication in motion." There is growing evidence that this mind-body practice, which originated in China as a martial art, has value in treating or preventing many health problems. And you can get started even if you aren't in top shape or the best of health.

In this low-impact, slow-motion exercise, you go without pausing through a series of motions named for animal actions — for example, "white crane spreads its wings" — or martial arts moves, such as "box both ears." As you move, you breathe deeply and naturally, focusing your attention — as in some kinds of meditation — on your bodily sensations. Tai chi differs from other types of exercise in several respects. The movements are usually circular and never forced, the muscles are relaxed rather than tensed, the joints are not fully extended or bent, and connective tissues are not stretched. Tai chi can be easily adapted for anyone, from the most fit to people confined to wheelchairs or recovering from surgery. Health.harvard.edu

Trager Psychophysical Integration

Trager Psychophysical Integration is a movement therapy in which practitioners apply a series of gentle, rhythmic rocking movements to the joints. They also teach physical and mental self-care exercises to reinforce the proper movement of the body. The intent is to release physical tension and increase the body's range of motion. An example of Trager Psychophysical Integration as CAM is using it to treat chronic headaches.

Yoga

The word yoga comes from Sanskrit, an ancient Indian language. It is a derivation of the word yuj, which means yoking, as in a team of oxen. In contemporary practice, this is often interpreted as meaning union. Yoga is said to be for the purpose of uniting the mind, body, and spirit. How can this union be achieved? *Meditation is one way, but sometimes it is necessary to prepare the body for meditation by stretching and building strength. This is the physical practice of yoga, also know as asana.*

Most modern yoga practices rely heavily on the Yoga Sutras of Patajali, a series of aphorisms written c. 250 CE, as the basis for their philosophies. Patanjali classifies asana as one of the eight "limbs" of yoga, the majority of which are more concerned with mental and spiritual well-being than physical activity. Yoga.about.com

Spiritual energy is who we are and any of the above mentioned modalities are a way for us to become more in tune with our energetic self. We can become attracted to any of them or simply experience energy in our world in our own personal way. Many of the techniques above work on our energy field to create balance and harmony. They are also a way to experience healing, but healing is something that we own for our-self and it cannot be given to us by another person. Without our complete participation there is no healing.

There is no way that energy healing will work for anyone, if they negate it's ability to do so. Having an open mind and a willingness to try something to see for yourself if there is any healthy effect is a big plus. But just as any of the above modalities adjust our energy body to that which is healthier, we can also with the power of our thoughts, deny that they give any benefit or affect Any form of thought that we entertain, within our mind, delivers the results to our reality, so if we deem something as ineffective, it will be so for us.

Chapter 5

The Vibration of Healing

The spirit energy for healing that an energy practitioner uses is one that is simply open to the flow of benevolent life source energy with the underlying intention of their doing good works.

Let's answer a few provocative questions.

Can anyone do vibrational healing?

I believe that anyone can but it is also necessary to point out that certain levels of vibrational existence are so blocked with denser vibrations that the finer light energy vibrations of higher conscious existence do not flow freely through such a field. Usually a person who seeks the help of an energy practitioner has already committed to an understanding of what the energy worker does and therefore has bought themselves to a level of awareness and acceptance that a vibrational adjustment will occur. They have essentially accepted that healing is possible and have engaged in the process in order for it to become realized.

Can someone shift their own energy blocks?

You most certainly can shift your own energy-blocks but it is easier achieved with the help of someone tuned to the vibrations of your field and who can quickly assess what is causing your energetic block.

Find someone geared toward helping you to master and clear your own energy field and who just employs guidance and coaching and not a guru who expects you to follow verbatim what they tell you.

Only you can know what is right for you. The more you listen to your own inner guidance the clearer the message becomes.

If you treat your conflicts as opportunities for self-reflection and growth any dense energy is automatically bought into the open, so that you can choose a God like way to interact with it.

You are more spiritual than physical and your greatest power comes when you engage in life from that spiritual perspective. To heal, is to bring your spirit essence into your physical existence/experience.

Should an energy healer attempt to dissolve all energy blocks?

The training of most energy practitioners imparts that energy because of its powerful effect on someone's physical life will only be altered when the client is ready to let it go. I agree a healer can shift the vibrations of an energy field and alter energetic states but that may last as long as it takes before the client reconnects with whatever caused the block in the first place. Energy work occurs such that truly a practitioner should work with a client over some time to bring them slowly but surely to an understanding of their own part in the healing process. Without the self-care needed for one's state of health any energetic alteration by energetic means of another person may not have longevity.

What can we expected when an energy block is shifted?

Often an emotional release occurs and the client may find themselves crying or expressing/feeling emotions that were buried. When beliefs are shifted, an Aha! moment occurs and awareness expands giving a sense of clarity as new ways of thinking are then realized. Often in the body a person will feel a sense of lightness due to this clarity and even added strength and agility. Clarity, in regards to the dynamics of a relationship, occur with a person being able to clearly see how someone is draining their energy and what if anything they can do from that point forward to stop that from occurring.

Is an energy block ever beneficial?

All energy blocks serve a purpose, they point to the resistance we harbor against expressing the higher vibrational energy that we have available to us. This energy permeates all life and elevates all life. A block shows clearly our misalignment with the best expression of our self. And yet, it is because of a block that we gain in awareness and growth and through the process of shifting and re-patterning the underlying cause of the block, we learn new ways to live our days.

Where does a healing vibration come from?

The vibration of healing is a vibrational frequency that you have access to. Simply put you can direct your own healing as many people have done. If you are ready to take on the task of self-healing it does not mean that you have to do it alone but what it does mean is that you understand that you are able to connect with a divinely inspired power within you and can then bring it forth to effect changes in your physical well-being.

Not all people are able to release the paradigms of their youth and especially the collective teaching that it is necessary to visit a doctor for healing. It is not beneficial for a person who strongly believes in this , to attempt self-healing; until their beliefs which govern their existence are reassessed for their continued validity.

Why do my physical symptoms keep appearing?

You are still holding an energetic alignment with the physical symptoms so that they keep up their appearance. If you become aware of the vibration that created the physical symptom then you can discover the belief or experience that created it and alter its effect on you then the physical symptom also alters.

How can I be healthier?

When you *seek* health you send a message that you do not have health in this moment you put *health* in the place of you not having it now. When you ponder a physical ailment then you strengthen its place in your life now. You may have an unconscious belief that states that at a certain age you will experience certain health issues. In which case you put yourself into a place of expecting that outcome. When you can over ride this belief that certain health issues must appear at a certain age then you can overcome the belief by looking at how people today actually live longer and healthier lives. It is completely within your energetic power to decide what health state you will experience in your life. Especially after you recognize and give up any generalized programmed beliefs you took on as a child.

The vibration of healing, is whatever meaning you give to it. To heal self means that a perceived adjustment in health is necessary. If that is the case, then healing will occur because any adjustment or change will alter the reality you live. If that adjustment brings you joy then your reality improves, if the adjustment does not deliver joy then you will inherently readjust until you find your bliss.

You could spend a life time searching for whatever will give you whatever it is you think you want, such as health.

This is because you always see anything you want, in a position of, to be searched for. When you actually stop the searching and claim your health, you alter your dimension to living healthy in the *now.* Because when you live in the here and now, you do not have to search for health because you already have it.

Is searching for health a bad thing?

No, there is no judgment, only your experience in this reality and if you are searching for health then the experience is a vibration you are presently living. It is the path to discovering what you claim as your own state of health.

Why have healing modalities if we can just live our health?

Healing modalities are a form of energy work that promote maintenance of the energy field, They work at the unseen level of existence and for many this level is a new discovery. So energy modalities expand our awareness and involvement in the existence of unseen energy.

While people hold a dominant perception that there are boundaries to their physical existence, then they can only live life within those boundaries. Because of this they will only seek tangible cures for their health.

One of the most neglected or overlooked things that we can easily do to give us an immediate lift is to listen to music.

Music

Music has long been know to have an effect on the energy body and we all have that particular song that induces a state of peace and harmony. Children so readily take to music but as we age it seems that we put the music away in place of daily tasks. How many of us actually make time to just sit and allow the vibrations of the music to wash over us and bring our energy body to a harmonious resonance with that sound? Allowing ourselves to enjoy our own favorite music is a great adjustment to our energy body vibrations.

Sound therapy is now found as a very effective way to make changes to frequency of our energy body. Sounds are vibration and in universal Tao there are six healing sounds that you can do at home to effect specific areas of the body.

The Lung Sound

Fear is stored in the lungs. The lung sound transforms fear into courage.

Position: Sit on the edge of your chair with feet shoulder length apart. Place hands palms-up on your thighs. Raise both hands above your head, palms-up, with fingertips of each hand touching the tip of the other. Look up.

Lung sound: Place your tongue behind your closed teeth and, with a long slow exhalation, made the lung sound "SSSSSSSSSSS" (like the sound of steam from a radiator).

Visualization: Return your hands to the palms-up position on your lap and smile to your lungs. Imagine a white light shining upon your lungs, surrounding them. Concentrate on feeling the virtue (power) of courage.

The Kidneys Sound

The kidneys sound transform the emotional energy inside the kidneys into gentleness and generosity.

Positions: Sit on the edge of your chair with feet shoulder length apart. Place hands palms-up on your thighs. Lean forward and clasp your hands around your knees. Look up:

Kidney sound: Form an "O" with your lips as if preparing to blow out a candle. With a long, slow exhalation produce the sound "WOOOOOOOO."

Visualization: Return your hands to the palms-up position on your lap and smile to your kidneys. Imagine a blue light shining upon your kidneys, surrounding them. Concentrate on feeling the virtue (power) of gentleness and/or generosity.

Repeat two more times (a total of three), including the hands position and visualization.

The Liver Sound

The liver sound transforms the emotional energy inside the liver into kindness.

Position: Sit on the edge of your chair with feet shoulder length apart. Place hands palms-up on your thighs. Raise your hands palms-up over your head and interlock your fingers. Lean slightly to the left. Look up.

Liver sound: Place the tongue near the palate and, with a long, slow exhalation produce the sound "SHHHHHHHHHH."

Visualization: Return your hands to the palms-up position on your lap and smile to your liver. Imagine a green light shining upon and inside your liver, surrounding it. Concentrate on feeling the virtue (power) of kindness.

Repeat two more times (a total of three), including the hands position and visualization.

The Heart Sound

The heart sound transforms the emotional energy inside the heart into love, joy and happiness.

Position: Sit on the edge of your chair with feet shoulder length apart. Place hands palms-up on your thighs. Raise your hands palms-up over your head and interlock your fingers. Lean slightly to the right. Look up.

Heart sound: With the mouth wide open, exhale a deep breath slowly and produce the sound "HAWWWWWWWW."

Visualization: Return your hands to the palms-up position on your lap and smile to your heart. Imagine a red light shining upon and inside your heart, surrounding it. Concentrate on feeling the virtue (power) of love, joy and/or happiness. Know that the red light is burning away and transmuting any hatred emotion or self-pity into the virtue emotions.

Repeat two more times (a total of three), including the hands position and visualization.

The Spleen Sound

The spleen sound transforms the emotional energy inside the spleen into openness, fairness and justice.

Position: Sit on the edge of your chair with feet shoulder length apart. Place hands, fingers of each hand touching the others, palms-up, under your left ribcage. Inhale and with breath held, slightly push the sides of your hands in and slightly up, under the rib.

Spleen sound: While moving the hands under the ribs, place the tongue near the palate, and with a long, slow exhalation, produce the sound "WHOOOOOOOO" from the throat, like the sound of an owl.

Visualization: Return your hands to the palms-up position on your lap and smile to your spleen. Imagine a yellow light shining upon and inside your spleen and pancreas, surrounding them. Concentrate on the virtue (power) of openness, balance and fairness.

Repeat two more times (a total of three), including the hands position and visualization.

http://www.universal-tao.com/article/six_healing.htm

When a person's perceptional boundaries shift, their awareness expands, to let in new forms of health aid based more on the intangible but felt effect of working with energy. Until one shifts their perception to include embodying the real power of their own life and health, then health is as illusory as physical reality to a mystic.

It is always good practice to find time each day to feel your own energy-body vibrations. try to feel the specific areas that may hold low vibrations. Then do an energy clearing in this way:

Lay on a comfortable surface or sit in a chair and close your eyes

Take ten deep breaths and tune into your energy body.

Start at your feet and slowly move your awareness over your energy body, up to the point just above the top of your head.

You are just getting tuned into the subtle nature of your energy body, keep breathing in a natural rhythmic way.

Start at your feet again and remember that your energy-body is bigger than your physical body so when employing your awareness include an area about two feet from your physical skin.

Run this scan again and just be aware.

On the third time start at your feet and give attention to any denser or darker feeling energy areas.

Just become aware of them, take your awareness to just above the top of your head

Now, for the fourth time tune into your energy-body from the point above the top of your head and move down toward your feet, slowly move your awareness and hover at the point of dense dark energy.

Now ask the higher-self to shine the light of love to this area. You know this area is a sign of dense energy, that you may or may not know the reason for.

It is O.K. to not know why you have this denser energy because the vibrational energy from your higher-self will transmute this energy.

Thank your higher-self for sending love to the denser parts of your energy-body.

Your higher-self or casual body holds dominion over the energy body layers of physical, emotional, mental and etheric bodies. These layers are no longer supported by life source energy the moment you cross over from the physical realm. The causal body remains as store house for all that you spiritually gained while on earth.

If you suddenly or within an hour of doing this energy body healing; feel intensity of an emotion surfacing, it will be the shifting of the energy-block. If you feel like crying do so, any unexpressed emotion needs to flow. The vibration of love stimulates unexpressed emotions to flow and your energy-body regains the harmonious position of unity with the frequency of your higher-self.

Chapter 6

The Path of Your Personal Health

I have a couple of friends in their 90's, actually one of them is 96 and spending time with people who are more senior in age, has been a huge eye opener. The characteristics of these healthy active friends is easy to distinguish. One of the main traits is that they speak their truth; they just simply seem to have a decisive way that is not clear in some people. Their thoughts are based on years of experience and show they have a knowing that doesn't have to try anymore, it just simply is. They do not think in a double-minded way and are not just touting learned information but have developed healthy reasoning born of life long experiences of their own. I absolutely enjoy the way they guide, what, if any, medical attention in which they take part. This comes from the fact that they are in tune with their own body and how it speaks to them.

I also notice that they still have a willingness to discover and learn by asking questions and listening intently. Many healthy *Wellderly*, a term I heard at a local group, have a strong sense of humor. Here is a little example of that; one friend asked, if I could drive her to the local batteries plus store because she had five watches that no longer worked, because the batteries had expired.

We entered the store the day after Christmas and she handed over the quart size Ziploc bag to the tall blond male clerk and asked him to replace all the batteries. He walked into the back room and then returned and looked across the counter at my friend and said, "Today we are running a special on the lifetime warranty batteries, you can get them for $9.99 each as opposed to $10.99 or we have the regular batteries for $5.99 " my friend, without missing a beat, looked the young man in the eyes and said, "you can forget the special, because at age 93, I have no need for lifetime warranties, and I think the regular batteries will probably outlast me!"

I feel that we all can take a lesson from the book of Wellderly, and learn to become in tune with our own bodies in such a way that we decide when, where and how we balance harmonize and clear our energy-field so that we move through our days in the most optimum way possible.

How do we take all that is higher vibrational health and personalize it for ourselves? Because we do have to make it a personal journey in relation to maintenance of a healthy state in our own energetic field.

I feel that we can become so in tune with our own mind, and why we think as we do, our body and how it serves as a temple for our spirit presence and soul and how it is guiding our experience so that the energy which connects it all, is able to unify our multilevel presence. I also feel that as we embody more of this state of unification, that we then expand to knowing our self as a very functioning piece of the family of humanity.

So how is information in this book up to this point and the previous paragraph relevant to your own personal state of health? There are a number of things that you can begin to bring more definition to your own journey of health and they are as follows:

- Become more aware of the vibrational layers of your own body and how they speak to you.

- Learn how energy alchemizes and therefore manifests the world that you see before you.

- Recognize that certain surroundings are either going to elevate your vibration or act as a drain on your life source energy therefore lowering your vibrational frequency. This includes certain people who you interact with.

- Eat to elevate your vibration and I have found that by including foods from every color group which correlates with each of the energy gateways helps to maintain those gateways at an optimum state of vibration.

- Set yourself a set amount of time each day out in the vibrations of nature so that you become harmonized with the earth vibration and the healthy states of a unified collective Divine consciousness.

- Question the medical advice you may receive and ponder the holistic effect it has on your energy field. If a pharmaceutical has a long list of harmful effects is that something you want to add to your body?

- Increase your water intake each day so that you saturate your cells and allow energy vibrations to travel easier through your body.

- Eat non-GMO foods, and a more alkaline diet.

- Stop using the crutch of; other people know the solutions for your problems. Only we can truly intuit the correct solution to any problem we perceive.

- Introduce some form of aerobic movements or deep breathing technique into each day so that oxygen in the body is kept at a high level.

- Release any emotions when they are felt, this often correlates with speaking the truth in all situations.

- Learn something new every day to grow new neural pathways in the brain.

- Practice communion with the energy of your higher self, whether through meditation or in a creative artistic pursuit.

- Learn to accept and get along with others because the relationships that we have are the energetic connective points of a unified humanity.

- Practice gratitude everyday whether it be a person, a situation or just life itself.

- Know that we are all in this story and all valid as a very needed and valued expression of Divine spirit.

Only we can take responsibility for our internal projections. We have to know that we are worthy, we are deserving, of all that we wish because there is no-one greater than our unified self. We have to change our internal reality before we can change our external reality. When we take 100% responsibility of our own feelings and life we know that no one gave us a problem or caused a problem for us, we manifested all that we have, so that we grow toward being a unified spirit/physical self.

Many people who are in our lives provide for us our greatest lessons. No one has power over us unless we give them that power. If someone projects toward us a low perception of us then only we can say, *yes, it is true* or *no,*

I do not accept that. The more we know who we are the less someone can actually have a damaging effect on us.

All that we see is a projection of our vibrational content. We are in a relationship with everything around us because we have resonance through co-creation of everything that we see. We are not a victim when we have co-created the world we live in. But we become a victim when we give up our co-creative power and follow the story and promptings of other people that we meet.

Think about it this way, we as the person in the mirror, either know that as we move the reflection follows us or we have to pay attention to the reflection and try to follow its every move. One is a form of movement with effortless ease and the other is movement of great stress. Only we can know as we look out from our own perception to the world that we see if we are leading what we see being reflected back to us or are we following every push and pull, every whim and movement of others and our environment.

In fact our world is co-created from our projections by our thoughts. This is powerful because when we know that we, as one with God, have the power within us for Divine manifestation, then we also know that we are more suited to lead in our own life story and not follow the story of another persons invitation, unless we decide the invitation is one that is resonate with where we want to go.

When we accept that we can fully embody our God-self spirit-energy our body, mind and spirit, as three, become engaged in unison. The power of this harmonic unity elevates the frequency of our thought and physical biological process so that we send forth more of a higher spiritual vibration. The effects of this type of energy moving out of our perception causes a quicker manifest time than one we could of previously attained.

This is particularly powerful when it comes to healing and our power of transforming our state of ill-health through healing into a state of health. Only when we join with the infinite potential of our intelligent God-self do we express the power of instant healing, over what we see as a reflection of ill-health in our reality.

Relationships

Our relationships are the biggest way that we communicate the signature vibration that we keep. They are also the best way for us to practice forgiveness and compassion, but not all relationships are beneficial and just because we entered into a relationship with someone it does not mean that we have to stay in it, especially if it is keeping our vibration in a low serving state.

When you take a general look at your relationships are you happy with what you see most of the time? Do you have a healthy give and receive interaction going on with the people with whom you find yourself engaged. Or do you have some energy leaks or blocks going on, such as, do you feel resentful that certain people only come to you when they need a boost to their own energy. Do certain people expect too much and give nothing in return.

Having any form of low vibrational reaction, because of the presence of a particular person, keeps your energy body frequency low. In order to change your reaction ask, is there a way to look at that relationship or interaction from another perspective? Can you bring your own judgment about what is going on, to a healthier place? If a relationship issue is a problem due to something that happened in the past, is it something that you can let go of in this moment. Can you forgive and move on to send this person heartfelt love. Some simple ways to release the binds of low energy connections with others is to meditate and mindfully send forgiveness, just as you use your mind to pray. Send the person love and release them from any bind to have to apologize for anything that transpired between you.

Honor their role in your life as one that came to teach you a lesson, as from every interaction we have with another we can find the lesson we learned or were supposed to learn if we just look for it.

If you need to do something more than a mindful act, write how you feel as if you were talking to the person. Explain to the person how you feel and again forgive and send love for their continued success in the world and offer them a save and happy journey. You do not have to give them the writing unless you want to. They will receive the message, in due time, from the subtle energy motion that moves and connects all humanity.

If the effect of you interacting with a person has any form of physical, emotional or mental abuse, think about why you stay in a place to receive this. Any form of dysfunction in a relationship stems from our relationship with our inner-self.

If you are in an abusive relationship then reach out and ask for help, you are worth more than being on the receiving end of any abuse. But only when you decide that you are.

I lived on the receiving end of abuse for many years and can tell you there is a definite energy shift needed to never again experience abuse. If we keep our energy-body vibration at the level that says, *I am unworthy,* then we become unworthy of even the basic levels of healthy living and that includes living without violence.

I am not saying any of us deliberately want abuse but I am saying, only *you* can set the boundaries to empower yourself higher than the level at which abuse happens.

This unworthy vibration may have been an imprint from an early childhood experience and we have to rise above it. If you separate from an abusive partner, do some work on yourself with an energy healer before you get back into another relationship. Spend time in meditation and face the source of your insecurities and low self-worth because, not until you shed divine light on them can they truly be transmuted. If you do not do the work you simply repeat the cycle.

Most of our relationships aid us toward unifying with our higher-self. The more we are unaffected by negative dynamics of any particular relationship the more we step into our power. Many of us enjoy the intimacy of having a romantic relationship. We enter the relationship with dreams of romance, kindness, giving, loving, we never for a moment consider the energy of that other person and what could be ripe to appear. As two energy-fields come together they harmonize as one. The denser energy of either of the two will shift and surface so that both people will share in its appearance. Are you flexible enough to understand that your lover may not have come to the table with an empty backpack? What if the nagging low vibrations of his secret financial issues, surface six months into your relationship or the fact, he is still emotionally connected to every girlfriend he ever dated and operates with an energy-body filled with past issues and old-time hurts. Can your energy vibrations remain high and unaffected in this particular close relationship. Remember in any close encounter you are now *one* and whatever issues he/she has, so do you. It amazes me sometimes when I hear from people, that an intimate act with another will not leave a lasting impact on their own energy-body. Hey, if you have sex with someone you mingle with their energy-body vibrations just as they become affected by yours. So before you go intimate with another, make sure you want to deal with any issues they struggle with, as they will rear their ugly heads and you will deal with them at some point.

I am not saying the above so that you avoid relationships altogether but awareness empowers so we confidently, compassionately and empoweringly deal with whatever transpires in our life. Sometimes surprises derail any spiritual gain that we have attained.

When we engage with other people and their issues no longer trigger energetic denseness, we as a detached observer, are able to offer inspiration from our place of power.

Whatever shows up as an issue in a relationship, is the reflection of an aspect of our own being, which needs some work. We cannot blame another for what happens in our life and stay in an empowered state. Just as we cannot blindly follow others over guidance of our higher-self.

Over fifteen years ago I experienced a continuous string of unexplainable physical symptoms. I reluctantly went to a doctor and received some pills that he said, I would take for the rest of my life. Somehow, this just didn't seem right to me. So, I handed him back the pills and said, "You take them for the rest of your life." Not long after that I heard guidance from my higher-self and lets just say, nothing remained the same in my reality since. My living arrangement changed and the pills were never needed.

Chapter 7

A Government View on Complementary and Alternative Medicine

Did you know that the government is now involved in the research and recommendations of Complementary and Alternative Medicine therapies to the public along with their research of traditional methods of medicine?

During my exploration of governmental views and research on Complementary and Alternative Medicine I came across a committee meeting dated, March 2000.

The meeting was well attended and shows how the government began its funding of research into Complementary and Alternative Medicine but of special interest is attendance of Dr. Andrew Weil who at that time was a prominent spokesperson for optimal health and listed as one of the most influential people in the year 1997.

Prepared Statement of Andrew Weil,

Mr. Chairman, Senator Harkin, and members of the Subcommittee, thank you for inviting me to testify this morning. For many, many years, I have been personally and professionally engaged in the very issue under consideration by the Subcommittee this morning.

I am encouraged by the level of interest Congress has shown in behavioral, alternative, and mind-body medicine. I would be remiss if I did not recognize the hard work Chairman Specter and Senator Harkin put into the fiscal year 2000 Labor, Health and Human Services, and Education bill. In strong and certain language, the Subcommittee recognized the importance of training physicians in integrative medicine.

This language underscores our responsibility to meet the needs of the rapidly growing number of consumers who are demanding a more healing-oriented system of healthcare.

Recent data indicate that nearly 50 percent of all U.S. healthcare consumers have sought alternative medicine in some capacity, creating the expectation that physicians should be knowledgeably guiding their patients through a course of treatment that is right for them.

We can do this by ensuring that physicians and other healthcare providers have access to appropriate levels of education and training in the valuable relationship between alternative and conventional medicine. This is the spirit of integrative medicine--maximizing the body's innate potential for self-healing by weaving alternative approaches into mainstream medicine.

With consumers' growing interest in a more integrative approach to healthcare and Congress' intent to fund integrative medicine education and training programs, allow me to share the unique and specific work we are doing at the University of Arizona to develop a model which best responds to these expectations.

The University of Arizona Program in Integrative Medicine was
established in 1996 with seven objectives:
(1) Establish integrative medicine as a new direction within academic medicine, not as a new specialty;

(2) Develop a new model of medical education and curricula for use by other medical institutions;

(3) Train physicians, pharmacists, nurses and other healthcare providers in the theory and practice of integrative medicine;

(4) Challenge physicians and other healthcare providers to commit to their own health and healing;

(5) Develop integrative medicine clinics as models for clinical education, patient care, and outcomes research;

(6) Research theories and methods of integrative medicine including effectiveness of new models of medical education; and

(7) Produce leaders who will establish similar programs at other academic institutions and set policy and direction for healthcare in the 21st century.

The mission of the Program in Integrative Medicine is to foster the redesign of medical education to incorporate the philosophy of integrative medicine. The Program developed a core curriculum which is adapted for its various educational components: the Fellowship in Integrative Medicine, the Associate Fellowship in Integrative Medicine (the ``distance learning" model for clinicians), Continuing Professional Education (CPE), pre-medical and medical education, and education of healthcare professionals.

It is important to note that this curriculum does not represent a linear process. Rather, curriculum components are interwoven to form an educational program that provides students, physicians and other healthcare professionals with a comprehensive education depicting the philosophies, principles and practices that are central to integrative medicine.

Philosophical Foundations.--The most fundamental distinction of integrative medicine is to shift the orientation of medicine from disease to healing. This requires students to closely examine their attitudes, not only with respect to medicine but also the manner in which they view the world. Courses include healing oriented medicine, the philosophy of science, medicine and culture, the art of medicine and research education.

Lifestyle Practices.--A basic principle of integrative medicine is that the manner in which we live clearly affects our health and disease. Lifestyle practices and prevention are central to this approach. This component of the curriculum focuses on the basic aspects of life and health that are addressed in the care of patients as well as practitioners of integrative medicine. Courses include spirituality and medicine, mind/body medicine, nutrition, and physical activity.

Therapeutic Systems and Modalities.--This component explores a variety of modalities and therapeutic systems. The history, theories, appropriate applications and scientific evidence are presented for each system and modality.

Physicians, healthcare professionals and students learn the techniques for some of these therapeutic modalities. More frequently, by presenting the theories and appropriate applications for these systems and modalities, those persons participating in the Program learn when and to whom they should refer their patients for the best treatment strategy individualized for their care.

Courses include botanical medicine, manual medicine, Chinese medicine, homeopathy, energy medicine, guided imagery and hypnotherapy.

The coursework described above, while often taught experientially, is content-oriented. The following are more process-oriented, and are not, therefore, broken down into specific courses.

Personal Development and Reflection.--Approaches involved in the practice of integrative medicine require practitioners to commit to their own process of self-exploration and personal development. The current methods used to educate medical students often result in the underdevelopment or degradation of these processes, and often translate into sub-optimal interactions with patients. This component of the curriculum is focused on methods for relaxation and self-examination of the healthcare professional. Included are such practices as meditation, personal reflection and group process.

Clinical Integration.--The process of integrating philosophically different systems of medicine into one comprehensive treatment plan for each patient is one of the most central features of the practice of integrative medicine. The goal is to teach the art of integration, not simply the strengths and weaknesses of alternative practices. In the absence of physicians or other healthcare providers who are educated and practiced in the art of integration, patients are torn between the instructions they receive from their conventional physicians, alternative care providers, health food clerks, the Internet, and their families in making their own medical decisions.

Healthcare providers must be skilled in understanding when and how to incorporate alternative approaches and to counsel patients against useless or fraudulent practices. This component also focuses on the integration of such philosophies and approaches into the practitioners' own personal and professional life.

Furthering the Field/Implementation.--This curriculum component is designed to help physicians and other practitioners put into practice what they have learned. There is strong focus on physicians as leaders functioning as agents of social change. Content areas include practical skills such as public speaking, business planning and management skills; social-political aspects of integrative medicine; medicine and law; and related ethical issues. For clinicians in practice, the emphasis is placed in putting this education into action within their clinical settings. This core curriculum serves as the blueprint from which specific curricula are designed to meet the needs of the various educational components of the Program in Integrative Medicine.

March 7th 2000, is in my mind a pivotal turn of events for, integration of conventional and alternative healthcare;

because it was on that date that President Clinton announced creation of the White House Commission on Complementary and Alternative Medicine Policy. The purpose was to study and report on public policy issues in the rapidly expanding field of complementary and alternative medicine.

Since then the Consortium of Academic Health Centers for Integrative Medicine was launched with a mission:

"to help transform medicine and healthcare through rigorous scientific studies, new models of clinic care, and innovative educational programs that integrate biomedicine, the complexity of human beings, the intrinsic nature of healing and the rich diversity of therapeutic systems"

For a medical education establishment to become a member they had to commit to develop a robust program in two areas: research, education, and clinical delivery of complementary and alternative medicine.

So, finally, healing practices which were before considered ineffective, and which were often ridiculed as *woo-woo* practice, making it difficult for them to be taken seriously are now getting recognition from the government, simply because these practices have grown in public demand, gaining mainstream status; on their own merit and without the need of the government.

So what does this show in terms of our responsibility for our own state of health?

It shows that we are no longer going to sit, listen and believe everything we are told about our state of health. It also means that we do have to learn to listen to our own body and have the confidence to act on what we intuit is the most beneficial way to return our unhealthy moment back to one of a healthy vibration.

This is positive, empowering and inspirational not only for us but for future generations. Because today we are actively making changes occur in the medical field that are more conducive to health and less conducive to creating lifelong patients.

Many of the active people I know in their 90's take very little if any pharmaceutical drugs. Surely this is a lesson for many of us. I have even heard first hand, elder patient's just flat-out say, "No," to their physician's recommendation, after which, they have engaged in choices suitable to them and have returned to a healthy state.

All of these are inspiring signs of what is yet to come. But they each contribute to one significant and powerful core paradigm, that we as a collective humanity are shifting toward responsibility of our own healthy state.

This is now reflected in the core values of the Consortium of Academic Health Centers for Integrative Medicine of which I say, are heartwarming and commendable;

Every person has the right to healthcare that:

- *provides dignity and respect*

- *includes a caring therapeutic relationship*

- *Honors the whole person-mind, body, and spirit*

- *Recognizes the innate capacity to heal, and*

- *Offers choices for complementary and conventional therapies*

I recently decided after five years of not going to a doctor to go and be thoroughly checked out before I embark on a year dedicated to maximizing healthy and healing vibrations. As an energy practitioner, mainly helping others raise their vibration mostly in the areas of renewing the mind, so they connect with inner spirit, I had decided to reintroduce Reiki to my practice. But before I did, I wanted to have that clean bill-of-health that scientific testing provides, just to corroborate my believe that I have a healthy energy-field and so I chose to visit a conventional doctor.

I am no spring chicken and am at an age when many women seem to experience slight aches, midlife conditions and undetected masses that if ignored could lead to dealing with bigger issues. I had not had a mammogram for ten years or an internal check of any kind. But I didn't see the need as I truly consider myself healthy, even if a little over weight. I also know that compared to the way I felt years ago I am of an extremely calm and happy disposition.

All of my tests came back as a healthy except for a thyroid issue that I had self-treated for over four years with Kelp.

Anyway, during that first visit with a new doctor to go over the tests and results I was absolutely taken aback. You see, this doctor was like none I had ever met before.

My previous visits to doctors had always left me feeling unheard, disregarded, and quiet honestly worse than when I entered their office. Most of the time, I left the doctor's office with a prescription for a drug I could not pronounce, little explanation of why I should take it and a vow never to return.

I must have acted on that vow, as it was not intentional that I did not go to a doctor for five years, but maybe there was a subconscious knowing that there was little if anything that made me feel better after doing so.

Anyway, at my first visit with this new doctor the discussion about my thyroid being low even though I was using Kelp was at the forefront. Kelp had helped for five years but it was obviously becoming less effective and was not providing the help my thyroid needed.

The discussion was going well but at the usual customary 15 minute mark of being with this new doctor I started to shuffle and picked up my bag in a gesture that I am ready to leave. This move was subconsciously enacted based on my experiences of previous visits to doctors.

This new doctor did not show any signs of reaching for the prescription pad or making final-notes that the visit was over. A few more minutes drifted by and so I said, "Thank you, I don't want to take up any more of your time I am sure you have lots of other patients to see," She looked at me and said, "Oh no, I do not, this is your time to see me and I have allotted an hour for this visit, how can I be of any help if I do not check you out thoroughly and answer all of your questions.?" I was literally dumbfounded. I put my bag down on the chair next to me and proceeded to talk.

I guess I did have some more questions about thyroid issues and when she couldn't off the top-of-her-head give those answers, she did what I have never seen before. She said, "wait here I will be right back," about two minutes later her tiny frame reentered the room carrying two huge blue medical encyclopedia. She said, "Just because I do not know the answers, doesn't mean we do not have a way of finding those answers." After thumbing through the books and letting me read along with her, my questions were answered and my perception of doctors was altered.

At about the hour mark after her entering the room, I honestly thanked her and said "I feel absolutely healthy as I leave your office today." She smiled and went about her day.

I feel this particular doctor is already providing the core values of the Consortium of Academic Health Centers for Integrative Medicine and others are sure to follow too.

Chapter 8

How a Non Genetically Modified Lifestyle Creates a High Vibe Energy Field.

When you grasp the power inherent within a person's intention and see it in action, revealing the fruition of its reward, it is a very rewarding sight.

I have a friend who around October, 2012 was the same size as myself. We were both a robust size 14, with desires to alter that appearance and move into healthier lifestyle.

We both had the typical symptoms of eating a Standard American Diet. Now known as S.A.D. and yes, I felt the usual lethargy associated with this diet which I believe also aids to a sedentary lifestyle. In fact many people in my life, who eat the considered normal American diet, have unhealthy lifestyles and unhealthy physical symptoms.

Anyway, my friend suddenly switched her lifestyle and diet so-much-so that I did not see her for almost a year. I continued my sedentary lifestyle, still eating the S.A.D but after my clean bill of health from a doctor and my wish to reintroduce energy healing in my daily work, I decided to alter my food intake and create a Chakra health diet. I was still developing and living those changes, when I received a pleasant boost from spirit. It came when I received and opened an email update from my friend. Included in that email update, was an inspiring health update. She had gone from a size 14 to a size 0 and had totally eliminated all GMO from her diet. This was something I was struggling to commit too, as well as my version of the Chakra health diet.

Her e-mail was a spiritual boost that I was on the right track with my diet changes and answered a question I had of whether to include a chapter on nutrition in this book. Really why even talk about health if we do not bring to light the food we use for physical fuel.

I am a chef and in our particular British training, I recall a heavy emphasis on the nutritional content of food. During my position as Executive Chef of Sarasota Memorial Hospital I gained experience in therapeutic diets and developed formed food for dysphagia patients.

I have previously been vegetarian, drank a diet of mainly juiced foods and dabbled in eating only raw food. The healthiest time of life was when I ate vegetarian and it was the diet-style that I thoroughly enjoyed.

But over the years, I admit while working to change careers from a job with a paycheck to total reliance on writing to pay bills, I slipped back into eating processed food, mainly due to the convenience factor, because it took less time away from my writing to just grab something and eat at the computer. Because of this, my energy to live an active lifestyle was also diminished.

Included in my friends e-mail update was the link to the Genetic Roulette Video. I highly recommend that anyone who is interested in genetically modified food watch this movie.

While I am not usually the type of person to put my attention on topics that I consider fueling fear vibration this movie just simply stated the facts about how our genetically engineered food creates changes in our genetics. While I watched the movie I felt a clear connection to my weight, health and sedentary lifestyle issues and the foods that the movie was talking about.

Needless to say my diet is now not only geared toward healthy Chakras but also toward absence of all genetically modified organisms. I truly believe that when we make a small shift toward a better way of life and make that change on both an inner or outer level the resulting shift in energy vibration draws to us more of what we want and therefore, also that which is needed for our continued expansion.

The receipt of the movie was a natural progression for my already attentive focus on what I am feeding my body at this time, in order for it to stay in a healthy disposition. My shift toward less processed and more vegetables made me look at not only the amount of vegetables but also the quality.

Why are GMO's something that we should consider avoiding? Genetically modified organisms alter foods, in such a way, that our body's immune system behaves as if it is under constant attack. This occurs because our immune system no longer recognizes food as food, because of its modified structure and toxicity. When we ingest foods, such as, meat, dairy genetically modified vegetables and fish that have either been treated with hormones or fed on genetically modified products, this form of nutrients necessary to build and repair our cells is now of a new genetic form . Our own genealogy is not aligned to processing these new forms of food, and as a result of that, our body performs in an unnatural and unhealthy way.

The way in which genetically modified food is altered is due to adding growth hormones and pesticides that alter the natural growth cycle of the plant or animal life. We are in essence forcing our control over nature and creating food that we, who are a product of nature, can no longer handle.

Growth hormones cross the digestive system into the genetic make-up of the human. I have personally noticed that I can no longer tolerate beef. If I eat beef my body immediately eliminates it and I also feel intense bloating and discomfort. After hours I notice an increase in joint pain and swelling, I just naturally eliminated beef from my diet.

All of these unnatural, additions to the physical layer of who we are also contribute in a huge way to our inability to become one with the inner layers of who we are. This is because we are creating an unnatural barrier, by way of altered genetics, that unfortunately bring on physical ailments and discomfort that grab our attention and keep it focused on what is wrong with us as.

While we battle bloating, discomfort, allergies, colitis, leaky gut syndrome, sluggishness, pesticide poisoning, allergies from the production and ingestion of these foods, we have our attention shifted onto those ailments. This is a clear hijacking of our energy and is simply a block and distortion in our energy field.

As we look at the way the body takes in, processes and uses the food we eat, we can also see that our digestive system is related to other physiological systems and if one system is fed in an unhealthy way, the others soon start to malfunction.

In America we have been increasing our use of processed convenience foods to the point where some people never actually eat naturally grown and harvested food. So what happens to the next inner system in the body when the first intake (digestive)system is fed with a substance that the natural biological code of the human body does not recognize? The next system, the immune system then goes into response and in an effort to ward of the invader (fake, altered, GM food) it is then activated and sends out the immune army to rid the body of these unnatural invaders.

Our immune response will now become compromised because it is biologically coded to ward off living organisms that want to infiltrate and take over the host (our body). These organisms include fungus, bacteria, molds, parasites, germs, viruses, but with GM, chemically processed and altered food, there are little real living organisms left in the food. So our immune system malfunctions because it is seeking the above mentioned living organisms and not finding any, it still recognizes that there are unnatural invaders within the body and the effort to remove them, is sent as a signal to the immune system as "failed."

So then our immune system ups the effort and the host (our body) has a continuous internal malfunctioning because the confused immune system, floods the digestive system and our body and we find that it attacks the cells of the host (our body) itself to rid the body of the invaders.

When our food has been given unnatural growth hormones and that food becomes ingested, the immune system recognizes which particular food, as in my case beef, triggers an immune response and because of the growth hormones associated and possibly similar to my own hormones, my body is constantly attacked in response to the food being eaten.

In the case of gluten, which is a member of the yeast family, the immune system is again set off, because gluten has also been genetically modified and the natural biological, digestive and immune systems , know that this is not normal food, but foreign substance, which does not belong and so the immune system attacks the invaders. More food ingested, more immune response, until the immune system is continuously fighting inside our body.

I am in no way a scientist, but have read, studied and determined from my experience, how my body reacts after I eat certain foods. I recognize the swellings, bloating and joint pain and while listening to my body, I now know that only I can stop putting these foods inside my body.

Will there come a day that genetically modified foods will be acceptable in a human biological system, because that system itself has been genetically altered by the mothers food intake in utero.? Or will food become so altered that we would be best served by learning to live on the energy of light?

There are people on the planet who survive and call themselves Breatharians. They have learned to live without ingestion of food and some even liquid. They use breath to receive Pranic life force and use this to stay in vitality and good health. This idea, while not new, is growing and worth keeping in our awareness radar, because it is now at the same stage of human attention that complementary and alternative medicine once was!

An interesting type of lifestyle which recognizes our emanation from light and energy of Source. Because of this, the belief that we can reembody the frequency of Source and live as that, is the concept within the lifestyle.

But for those of us now reading this book, if you are having any symptoms of lethargy, fatigue, sluggishness, bloating, joint pain, sinus issues, asthma, or allergies, and any form of immune dysfunction it may help you to adjust your diet and drop some of the toxins our S.A.D now include.

Our energy-body speaks to us and it has its own language. The higher-self that we all have access too, holds the intelligent energetic blueprint for our own state of wellness. As we come to clear lower dense energy from our energy-body we are opening the pathways or meridians to flow this higher intelligent energy through our systems. If we negatively alter the energy-field of our physical body, the intelligent energetic flow is no longer aligned to the state of our physical body and we are essentially cut off from our own inner higher guidance until we clear the field to hear that guidance again.

We are all inter-connected on the energy matrix of humanity and we deserve to live healthy, whether we find that way through choices frowned on by others or choices that are an inspiration to others. Our journey is one journey as a unified and collective humanity, lets makes it the healthiest that we can.

My removal of genetically engineered and genetically modified food occurred during the course of writing this book. It was inspired because a friend asked me for a ride.

Jan 8th I met with Andrea Page and Terry Ryan (slimhealthysexy.com) at our local Paneras. The intent for the visit was; Terry interviews Andrea on her successful weight loss story by eliminating genetically modified organisms from her diet. Here is the transcript of Terry's interview:

"Wow, was my reaction when Andrea walked into Panera's on Cattleman Road, Sarasota, FL. The last time I saw Andrea, she had lost about 20 pounds but she still had away to go. Now here she was, down to a size 0 and looking fabulous! Andrea had sent me an email to a link to the movie The Genetic Roulette, and I watched it and was just as outraged as she was by what the FDA and Monsanto are doing to our food supply. She had said in the email that she had lost a substantial amount of weight. So, she is health conscious and concerned about GMOs, just like me, so I called her and suggested that we get together over coffee at Paneras, our normal place to meet.

Here is my conversation with Andrea:

Me: What was the catalyst that motivated you to lose weight?

Andrea: I watched the move **Genetic Roulette** and got so mad at what Monsanto was doing to our food, that I just decided that I wanted to eat healthier. I was determined that Monsanto wasn't going to poison me. All of my family is gone, they all died young and I am determined to live longer than them. I want to live until I am 150. (That is not a typo.)

Me: What was a typical day for you?

Andrea: (She hands me a flyer that she has made.) Breakfast consists of smoothies made with a **Bullet** (mixer). Everything is organic (of course), lots of fruits, nuts, dates, maple syrup for sweetness. Lunch and dinner is veggies such as tomato, red onion, red bell pepper, red cabbage, avocados, cukes, kale, potatoes, miller, lentils, chick peas, garlic, ginger, mushrooms, onions. They can be prepared raw or steamed. Snacks are dehydrated apples and bananas.

I noticed that Andrea had a glass bottle of cloudy water with her. She said it was water and fresh squeezed lemon juice. She also had samples of her dried apples and bananas that she gave us that were very good. "I needed something crunchy to snack on so I make these," Andrea told us.

Me: So how much weight have you lost all together and when did you start?

Andrea: I have lost 60 pounds and I began October 2012. (Today's date is 1/8/2014)

Me: Did you make little changes or did you go full on cold turkey?

Andrea: Cold turkey.

Me: Did you crave anything or feel terrible when you started?

Andrea: No, I felt fine because I was already eating pretty healthy when I started. I did go to bed for the first week crying because I couldn't eat my bowl of popcorn at night.

From Andrea's Flyer:

This is how I started the switch, (I watched Genetic Roulette Movie, The World According to Monsanto.)

1. Dr. Oz Three Day Cleanse.

2. Two week Alkaline diet. ("Dropping Acid")

3. Rainbow diet – 100% Organic foods. (Basically means eating a lot of colorful veggies.)

4. Commit to non processed foods, and go vegan if you can, non-gmo and as much organic as possible. Eat "whole, fresh foods."

5. Clean your liver first thing in the morning with lemon in your water in place of coffee.

6. Also read **Natural Cures** by Kevin Trudeau. Great info.

Me: Kevin Trudeau as in the guy who ran to Switzerland to avoid paying taxes?

Andrea: Yes, he has a lot of good information in the book.

Me: What do you do when you go out to a restaurant?

Andrea: I bring my own food.

Me: What? No, that's not possible. Really, what do you do when you go out to dinner with friends.

Andrea: I don't go out to eat.

Me: That would be a big problem for me and my friends who like to go out to eat.

Andrea: Yeah, that would be tough, I agree, but I don't go out.

Me: Do you ever go off the diet and eat a hot fudge sundae?

Andrea: No never. Do you know what is in dairy?

Me: Yes. (Bovine growth hormone, antibiotics, etc.) What about organic milk?

Andrea: I don't really trust that it is organic.

"I'm passionate about removing all the toxins from my body and my life. My goal is health and longevity."~Andrea Page

Me: Do you use a sugar substitute like Stevia?

Andrea: I don't really trust that either.

Me: Health wise do you feel any differently?

Andrea: I no longer have migraines, my knees don't hurt anymore, and my skin is clearer.

Me: Did you notice anything else?

Andrea: My taste buds reset after 90 days where I no longer had any cravings or desire for sweets or other non healthy food.

We finished our conversation ended it with what Andrea was up to with her business with Send Out Cards and we agreed to meet on Thursday (1/16/2014) at Tanya's house to clean out all the junk food and go shopping for organic veggies. I'm bringing the video camera and will be recording the entire process.

More to come...

http://www.slimhealthysexy.com/from-size-14-to-0-andreas-story/

This above meeting was a synchronistic event in action, the universe could not have played it any clearer, because I had just finished writing *Higher Vibrational Health* and during meditation I requested more content to inspire and encourage I had written a small section about GM food. But little did I know that section would expand in my life to become a year-long commitment.

I was writing about vibrational health but quite honestly I was not living at my healthiest vibration and I knew it, but that was about to quickly change. During the course of conversation after Terry's interview I heard myself offer to follow the developed way of Andrea so she could market *her way* to help other people.

I left the meeting with an appointment for Andrea to come to my home and for Terry to film the raid of my kitchen and let me know just how much of a toxic pantry I harbored.

I decided not to fake it, I could have thrown out all the toxic stuff and made it look like I was somewhat healthy before she came to visit. But I was not the only one eating from the food supply in my house. My 17-year-old when not visiting friends and my 11-year-old daughter ate there and they would not take kindly to finding only vegetables in the cupboard.

I had actually started adjusting my food intake around October last year when I visited the doctor. This was because after a series of tests and visits that proved my healthy state, a doctor said to me, "next visit we will tackle your weight." I looked at her and said, "what lose weight!" she looked at me and said, "Yes." So as the next visit was coming to an end, I thought, ask about the weight loss comment that she mentioned during the previous visit. So I said, "last visit you talked about dealing with my weight issue,' I was thinking that she was going to give me the magic pill, you know, the one you take, exert no effort and bam the 45Ibs are gone. She looked at me and said, "Oh yes! Eat less, move more!" While this was not what I was hoping to hear, it was exactly what I needed to hear. I know there are no magic pills and agree that I need to move more, as writing is one of those sedentary lifestyles, that easily produces weight gain, if not balanced with activity.

I started by increasing my vegetable intake so that I could balance my Chakras. This increase in vegetables was going well but it was the underlying staples of food, coffee and sugar consumption that I really needed to adjust. So for now coffee and sugar were out and non GMO was in. I was going to do it *The Andrea Way* until I felt confident that I could go it alone. I had no coffee or sugar the day of the interview.

Here is an account from my diary of shifting from genetically modified food to an organic food intake.

Jan 9th I woke with a headache and an extreme craving for sugar I resisted the temptation by having a cup of ginger peach tea. I was hungry and sent a short email to Andrea to ask if tea was toxic, she recommended that I use tea leaves acquired from the organic food shop. I was not in the mood to go out but luckily I had received two bags of tea leaves at Christmas. I didn't know if they were organic but they would have to do until I got some.

Food consumption: two pouched eggs, strawberries, half a cantaloupe melon, bowl of homemade vegetable soup, two cups of tomato juice.

Thank God my daughter was at her father's house that evening because I was in no shape for anything, the headache raged and I lit a candle, put on some light music and lay on the couch. Tossing and turning till I went to bed.

January 10th Woke up at 10.30 am feeling a little better today but the headache is still there it is fading in intensity I suddenly remembered that years ago I fasted every Friday and would reintroduce a *fasting* day but today would not work as I felt I needed to eat something. Again I didn't have any lemon and didn't feel like going out so I substituted lime for the lemon until I went organic food shopping.

I received a text response to a question I asked my son Tyson about weight he was lifting . He said, " 515 lbs" I sent him a text about my healthy choice for 2014, not sure if I was trying to compete with the 515lbs, but giving up sugar and coffee certainly felt as if I was. He sent a text back that said,. "The most important thing is consistency you have to stick with it when it gets tough. The results will be slow just stay positive and mentally strong. You can do this," and so it is, that day three of GM and sugar detox continues with a slight headache and some positive inspiration.

By 2.00 pm my headache had increased and I once again relegated myself to the couch until I had to pick up my daughter. That evening I had a dinner invitation but canceled because I was not up to it. I left the house to pick up Avalon with her father and we stopped at The Blue Rooster in Sarasota for a drink. I chose Bloody Mary as the least alcoholic with the most vegetables. For some reason the drink did not appeal to me, so I drank half. Later we went for a bite to eat, this was a big test, as I had to scour the menu for healthy food, I settled on Tilapia, zucchini, squash, and broccoli, with herbal tea. I declined the invitation for dessert, although temptation was strong. I went home and laid down.

Food consumption: two boiled eggs, fish, zucchini and yellow squash, broccoli, one small orange, quarter of cantaloup melon, three bottles of water.

January 11th Woke up without a headache, woke up feeling invigorated and raring to go, so set to cleaning the house. I as a coffee lover am investigating to find a coffee that is organic, my husband suggested Green Mountain coffee, because Vermont does not allow pesticides to be used in their state.

I started the morning with a bottle of water and a cup of tangerine tea, it was a tea bag, something Andrea said to avoid but I will slowly use up what I have in my closet and intermingle it with the tea leaves. I will do a little investigation to find if Celestial Seasonings tea would pass as organic as I believe they are also from Vermont.

Here is a definition of, Genetically engineered, according to Vermont statures:

"Genetically engineered (GE) seed" means seed produced using a variety of methods, as identified by the National Organic Program of the U.S. Department of Agriculture, used to modify genetically organisms or influence their growth and development by means that are not possible under natural conditions or processes. Such methods include cell fusion, microencapsulation and macroencapsulation, and recombinant DNA technology (including gene deletion, gene doubling, introducing a foreign gene, and changing the positions of genes when achieved by recombinant DNA technology). Such methods do not include the use of traditional breeding, conjugation, fermentation, hybridization, in vitro fertilization, or tissue culture.

(10) "Genetically engineered plant part" means a whole plant or plant part, including scions intended for planting, which contains material derived from a GE seed or is itself produced using the methods described in subdivision (9) of this section. (Added 1989, No. 85, § 2; amended 1989, No. 256 (Adj. Sess.), § 10(a), eff. Jan. 1, 1991; 2003, No. 42, § 2, eff. May 27, 2003; 2003, No. 97 (Adj. Sess.), § 2, eff. Oct. 1, 2004.)

http://www.leg.state.vt.us/statutes/fullsection.cfm?
Title=06&Chapter=035&Section=00641

"More than 20 years ago, Senator Leahy first became involved in the organic movement because he had heard from many Vermonters that there was a significant market for high quality farm goods produced in an environmentally friendly manner. They were right. The organic industry is the fastest growing sector of American agriculture, and it is especially strong in Vermont. Vermont boasts the highest number of certified organic farms and certified acreage per capita in the nation, as well as hundreds of businesses producing and selling value added organic products.

Senator Leahy realized early-on that the organic revolution would only be possible if "organic" really meant something that consumers could understand and trust. That is why he wrote the Organic Foods Production Act, which passed as part of the 1990 Farm Bill and created strong and credible federal standards so that now, over twenty years later, consumers know what organic means. He has pushed the Department of Agriculture to ensure the designation "organic" signifies that a product is not genetically engineered and is grown without the use of synthetic fertilizers or pesticides."

https://www.leahy.senate.gov/issues/agriculture-nutrition-and-dairy

Went to the local coffee shop this morning ordered water and a Greek yogurt parfait 15 gram protein with granola and honey. It looked healthy until I saw the sugar content. Wow! 30 grams . I read the ingredients which also seemed healthy enough including pumpkin seeds, and rice flour and coconut but the taste was definitely way too sweet and so I passed it over to my husband.

Came home and ate some home-made vegetable soup.

Went to Richards a local health shop for a snack item, I looked at the rows of dried food dispensers and settled on sultanas because they only had one other ingredient listed. I was in a health food shop, so trusted the label but still researched on the internet that other ingredient; sulfur.

Imagine my chagrin when a Google search showed negative and allergic effects to consuming food with sulfur Some effects include; breathing problems such as asthma, emphysema, chronic bronchitis, and respiratory disease. When eating foods treated with this gas, some may experience skin rashes, an upset stomach, or an asthma attack. Not exactly what I had in mind when I went into the health shop to buy a snack.

More trusty home-made vegetable soup and off to the shop tomorrow to buy some organic fruits to see if I can dehydrate them in the oven. No I do not have a dehydrator yet but am working on getting one.

Food consumption: ½ Greek yogurt parfait, bottle of water 20oz, 2 cups of home-made veg soup, one boiled egg, one clementine, 2 cups of tomato juice.

January 12th woke up feeling great, feel as if I am no longer detoxing. I made a cup of lemon detox tea which seems to have become my favorite choice for morning tea, and ate a fried egg and clementine for breakfast.

Today my research was on honey, I love honey due to its sweetness and because I have always considered it a super food and healthy for humans.

I unearthed that honey is good for us but honey along with other foods has fallen prey to mans interference and because of its filtration most of the honey now found on our local grocer's shelf is no more than sugar. Why is that so? Well for honey to be honey it needs to have pollen in it. It is the pollen that includes the health benefits. Most of our honey is highly filtered and no longer has the benefits of organic honey.

The benefits found in raw honey come from the pollen. They include:

"**1. Energy Enhancer** -The range of nutrients found within bee pollen makes it a great natural energizer. The carbohydrates, protein and B vitamins can help keep you going all day by enhancing stamina and fighting off fatigue.

2. Skin Soother -Bee pollen is often used in topical products that aim to treat inflammatory conditions and common skin irritations like psoriasis or eczema. The amino acids and vitamins protect the skin and aid regeneration of cells.

3. Respiratory System -Bee pollen contains a high quantity of antioxidants that may have an anti-inflammatory effect on the tissues of the lungs, preventing the onset of asthma.

4. Treating Allergies –Pollen reduces the presence of histamine, ameliorating many allergies. Dr. Leo Conway, M.D of Denver Colorado, reported that 94 percent of his patients were completely free from allergy symptoms once treated with oral feeding of pollen. Everything from asthma to allergies to sinus problems were cleared, confirming that bee pollen is wonderfully effective against a wide range of respiratory diseases.

5. Digestive System -In addition to healthful vitamins, minerals and protein, bee pollen contains enzymes that can aid in digestion. Enzymes assist your body in getting all the nutrients you need from the food that you eat.

6. Immune System Booster -Pollen is good for the intestinal flora and thereby supports the immune system. According to holistic health expert Dr. Joseph Mercola, bee pollen has antibiotic-type properties that can help protect the body from contracting viruses. It's also rich in antioxidants that protect the cells from the damaging oxidation of free radicals.

7. Treats Addictions –Used holistically for healing addictions and inhibiting cravings by suppressing impulses. Because bee pollen crashes cravings, it is a very useful research is needed into this benefit, particularly when it comes to weight management.

8. Supports the Cardiovascular System -Bee Pollen contains large amounts of Rutin; an antioxidant bioflavonoid that helps strengthen capillaries, blood vessels, assists with circulatory problems and corrects cholesterol levels. Its potent anti-clotting powers could help prevent heart attack and stroke.

9. Prostate Aid -Men who suffer from benign prostate hyperplasia can find relief by using bee pollen. Bee pollen can help reduce inflammation to stop frequent urges to urinate.

10. Infertility Problems -Bee pollen stimulates and

restores ovarian function, therefore may be used to assist in accelerating pregnancy. As-well-as being a hormonal booster it is also a great aphrodisiac!"

http://foodmatters.tv/articles-1/10-amazing-health-benefits-of-bee-pollen

I finally went shopping and loaded up with organic vegetables and decided to cook a nice diner that night. I checked some of the usual products I buy, like hummus and quickly returned them to the self when I could not pronounce some of the ingredients. I bought the ingredients to make my own hummus.

Food consumption: collard greens, pistachio nuts, broccoli, sweet potato, blackberries, three bottles of water, water with lemon, three cups of tea

January 13th I awoke feeling as if I finally have food in a proper perspective of nourishing my physical body. My mind is very alert and clear. I feel energetic and highly focused on my goals for this day.

Enjoyed a 32 oz bottle of water, and drank my detox lemon tea with milk thistle and lemon verbana.

Was just informed by a friend of mine that I can get honey with pollen from the neighboring town.

Food consumption: banana, half a sweet potato, three cups of hot tea, bowl of home-made soup (includes potato, collard greens, red onion, carrots, celery), boiled egg

Today I contemplated why we eat and the relationship between our health and food consumption. Can foods with a higher vibration quickly elevate our energy field? By only ingesting those type of foods and eliminating processed or genetically engineered foods can we alter the type of thoughts we have and the emotions that we feel? Can we alter our signature vibration?

After only five days of a complete food overhaul I honestly feel clean, light and more in tune to my biological make up.

I have not experienced any of the intermittent stiffness or joint swelling/pain since the food switch and am looking forward to remaining agile. While I believe that disease comes because of an underlying cause and a distortion in our energy-field, it may for some people be as simple as the food eaten, causing that distortion.

Chapter 9

How To Raise Our Energy Vibration Today

We all give away our ability to receive from the highest purest clearest vibrational frequency that there is, when we invite the energy vibrations of other people's past experiences, out-dated beliefs, cranky moods and low emotions to take up residence in our energy field.

We also do so when we engage with memories because memories alter perception and take us back to what-ever we are remembering. A life truly lived in the present moment does not play in the realm of memories.

While the Source of creation always emanates the best light energy to sustain us, we do have ability to allow subconscious conditioning to override that energy. How long will we do this; for as long as it takes us to discern what is right for us? Are we going to hear the guidance and receive the light or are we going to keep our attention on the external experiences and try to alter life by altering them?

In almost any situation in which we find challenges, there are along with that challenge, great lessons learned so that we do not manifest those particular challenges again.

But those challenges are not originally of a physical manifestation but born of an inner energetic projection. It is this that may take a little while to grasp, as we have been taught that life is only what we see and not what it actually is and that is; what we create.

Nature is unhurried and if it takes a lifetime for us to see the cycle of life and how we create what happens, so we can make a change and not repeat what we do not want to experience again, then so be it. Sometimes the most *shifting* lessons are the ones that take a while to learn.

If we look at the reflection of creation we can do so with this in mind, when we see life with our physical eyes, it means we see life from two, meaning we see life in a state of duality. When we see life from our spiritual eye, or our third eye, it means we see life as one, meaning in a unified state.

Now that many people have grown in understanding about energy and vibrations and are viewing life more from unification of spiritual sight, we all readily see the tools and knowledge to quickly shift any challenge into a golden opportunity of *lesson learned and lifestyle changed.*

Often the situations where we halt the higher energy flow that wants to appear in our life include;

- not giving to ourselves,
- doing work that we do not love,
- not speaking the truth,
- remaining in a relationship that is unhealthy for us,
- eating too much processed or GMO food,
- giving in to addictions,
- relying on pills to mask pain and depression,
- allowing past traumas to dictate how we live now,
- giving in to the demands of society as opposed to our inner wisdom,
- exercising double mindedness, and
- not being co-practitioner in our healthcare decisions...

...but they are easy to change. It might take a little help from an energy worker, preferably someone who is not presently enmeshed in the dynamics of our everyday life.

When you bring new energy vibrations into the energetic matrix of any situation, that situation has to alter. A person who is not enmeshed in your energy dynamics will also be in the clearer place to perceive that which you do not and to then offer an unbiased observation, after which, they can draw from within you, what it is you would like to change while they strengthen your ability to receive guidance from spirit.

When we get closer to living the life that excites us, we are in fact raising our energy vibration to one that is closer to our authentic essence. While we partake of this vibrational climb we will often suddenly experience negative situations. This can make it seem as if we are not making any real headway. But, there is a reason, when we set ourselves on a path of healthier lifestyle we find that difficulties arise. This is so, because, we at that moment have some buried content within our energy field. It could be in the form of subconscious beliefs or negative memories.

Lets look at the dynamics of that, often the reasons that we are presently making poor lifestyle choices are buried within the energy matrix of who we are. In order for us to grow into the lifestyle choice that we find healthier, the vibration of the poor choices, will have to shift and come up from their placement within our matrix so that they become altered. In doing so, we may once again experience or at least become aware of the reason behind the poor choices we make. At this point we either, choose to keep doing or alter the reason for our choices, that lead to our present behavior.

This re-experiencing of buried content, in order to clear it from our energy matrix, comes as a reflection, from the mirror of our reality. Should we have difficulty with choosing the correct foods to support a healthy physical body, we will find our-self in situations which require us to make new choices and we will find our-self in those situations often enough, so that the new choice is now unquestionably what we will continue to do. Until it has essentially become our new vibration.

In order to create the life that we really want we have to ask, are we doing what energizes us most in life. When we can do what energizes us we re-vibrate our field and this out-flowing signal from our energy matrix brings a response of, more choices that truly energizes us.

If we want a healthier lifestyle; one that we truly believe will give us true health as we know it. We have to know what true health means to us. This is where many people fall flat. They spend most of their time looking around at what everyone else is doing and they set off on the path of another person's idea and forget to blaze-the-trail of their own health. Yes, we may need encouragement and direction at the beginning of any lifestyle change but ultimately we know and are fully responsible for our own healthy state.

I used to lift weights. I used to run daily. I did this for many years and was extremely healthy at that time. Ask me now if lifting weights excites me and I will honestly tell you, "No." I am grateful for the experience of lifting weights but have evolved beyond finding this as something I wish to keep doing and so am now in the process, as too are many other people, of finding a form of exercise that arouses a passionate vibration. I believe that some form of exercise is a natural part of a healthy lifestyle. But am not going to do something that I no longer feel guided to.

Until I find what excites me; being the one thing that will over-ride my vibration of, *no interest in lifting weights* I am momentarily paused, in knowing, I do not want to lift weights and yet have no present replacement for that.

This occurs for a lot of people, I have friends who say they do not like to sweat. But many activities of a healthy nature cause the body to perspire. In order for those people to find a form of exercise that excites them they can try activities like swimming or Tia chi until they find one that fits with not sweating. This preponderance of a definite statement of what we do not want, *I don't want to sweat,* is actually a help because its purpose will guide us to what we do want.

My son Tyson and his girlfriend Ashley both enjoy weight lifting and working out at the gym. Tyson is a personal trainer and they are both very active and yet at the same time they also enjoy many social events similar to their generation.

When I discussed my book with them and asked for any comments they said "health means enjoying a balanced life some work and lots of play." They also said, "we notice when we go to the gym with the thought that this is hard, then it becomes hard, but when we go to the gym with thoughts that this is easy, then it becomes easy."

Has life changed, so that in an instant, life is now manifest on the spin of a thought. Has our collective ability to manifest, sped up, or is it the vibration of our younger generation who have a keener perception for the manifesting process than we do?

It is up to us to decide what will bring about a rise in our vibration. Our own unique way to carry this out is perfect for us.

But here are a list of actions to think about, to get your own creative juices flowing in regard to raising your own vibration.

Ten Ways to Clear Low Vibrations

1. "Think about, what you thinking about, when you are thinking it."

Thoughts are fabulous they are the building blocks of what we see. The world is a mirror of our thoughts and we live in an intelligent energetic universe. We can intuit and receive the intelligent expressions of our higher-self and we can transfer thoughts between the personal

Energy-Body's that we as a human share.

We receive the thoughts of our macro cosmic intelligence as we come to live our life more from our higher-level spirit body. The thoughts that we take on from, the usual avenues of media and other people may not serve us in our quest to realize life, from our authentic spirit presence within. Knowing that thoughts have such creating and manifesting potential we are well served to monitor our thoughts and as I like to say "think about what you are thinking about, when you are thinking it." This process will serve to bring you to a more aware state of the kinds of thoughts you are having and whether they are serving your growth toward the reality you wish to experience or are they hindering any forward movement for you and all others within this reality.

Only when you step outside a thought, are you in a stronger position to actually alter that thought. Assessing if our thought is human or divine; meaning limited or limitless gives you observation power to make a change.

Practice having divine thoughts because you are an expression of the Creator, so think like one.

2. **Use words that offer support, love and inspire other people.**

There are words that uplift sustain and inspire and words that tear down. We did not learn about the vibrational frequency of words in our schooling because little was known about the vibrational power of words, years ago.

If we look at a popular example of a way that many people talk to children, the phrase "Don't talk to me like that" sends an energy vibration of control and negativity. If we reword the phrase we can say "Please use a calm voice when we talk." Now we are sending an energetic vibration of request and gratitude. The energy vibration of each statement will be impressed upon the recipient of those very words.

The way that we use our words is one of the quickest ways to change our energetic frequency and that alone facilitates an upward shirt in energetic frequency. Making an effort to find other choices that express in a clear and considerate way our request of another, by removing demanding words such a don't, get, never and no, Our effort will be training our brain to seek alternatives and to intentionally look for a calmer more harmonious use of our words. Other word choices will appear naturally such as; please, can you, I feel like, etc. These are uplifting words, when we use them.

"Don't run"   "Walk please"
"Get me a drink"   "Can you please bring me a drink"
"I hate the movies" "I wish to go to the mall instead"

Knowing that words have an energetic frequency we can choose to consciously add empowering words into any conversation that we have with others. Words that offer our support and love or words that show we are in alignment with supporting success of other people can become a habit the more that we employ them. Such as
"I support you in your attaining that goal"
"I see for you much success with that project"
"That is a great idea I know you can be the one to make it happen."

When we consciously look for empowering, inspiring, uplifting words and infuse them into our daily communication, we add higher vibrational frequencies into our communication. The more we increase our vibration the quicker we transmute or clear out low dense content.

3. Forgive yourself and others for any perceived slight.

The act of forgiveness is powerful but it is not done in a way that we state that another has done us any wrong. When we forgive others we are acknowledging that we shared an experience with them but have now decided to let it go.

All life and situations are a shared moment with another person. Every single moment occurred due to our emitting an energy vibration that aligned us with that experience. We can, after that experience, keep residual effects in the form of, emotional blockages, non-serving beliefs or judgments within our energy field. Doing so, serves to have us repeat or re-experience, this similar content again.

When we forgive we are stating that it is time to let it go and we alter our energy-body vibration by releasing our attachment to any perceived slight.

Often we are harder on ourselves than we are on others, because we measure our-self against the standards of others in our world. This judgment blocks our authentic expression, as we try to live up to those standards. When we realize that there are only fluid standards, we see we are perfect the way we are. We are a valid member of the total consciousness of humanity and our authentic expression is what is unique and beautiful about our unifying with that total consciousness. We move to a place of acceptance and when others see that we are truly expressing without fear of their or our own judgment, they are then inspired by our authentic presence.

Each moment is a new moment, filled with love, beauty and the potential to co-create a fabulous existence. Living this way removes the need for guilt and eventually for forgiveness.

4. Express emotions as they occur.

Emotions unexpressed can stay within the emotional layer and cause havoc until processed and released; emotions exist and interpenetrate all the layers of the Human Energy-Body.

Emotions are usually a bodily feeling indicator of the experience you are having. Even if it does not feel so good, such as in the fear of public speaking it is beneficial to delve into the fear and find out why it is there. Fear of anything means it is still a vibrational frequency that you are choosing to entertain within your Energy Body.

Our Energy Body is emitting the vibration which then mirrors back to us as the contents of our reality. Only when we are one with fear can we change it. If fear is perceived as something happening outside of our own Energy Body vibrational field then we cannot possibly feel that we can change it, as we have given it an other-than-us state of existence. This means to make any change we would have to exert control over it. Exerting control over something will always keep it separate from us and therefore in that illusive state of never being able to be changed. Only that which we are unified with can be altered by us.

The processing of emotions itself can be difficult when we live in a world where "big boys don't cry." Denying emotional expression serves to maintain the energetic frequency of that emotion, as a long term resident of our own Energy Body.

Emotions show up in the body as physiological sensations like that flipping of your stomach when you are feeling indecisive.

To process emotions you simply experience them. To process buried emotions that resurface during an energy shift you can query what thought was attached to the energy movement and then work to change that thought. If you are faced with an emotional situation express it, as that is the purpose of our emotions, they allow us to be fully present in the moment and make choices based on what we feel.

Emotions provide awareness and are a healthy truthful expression. You do not just experience emotions; you can choose to have emotions.

It was a very empowering moment for me when I looked at the general emotions I engaged in, about a job I was not overly keen on performing. I consciously made a choice to not be defined by my emotions but to display a state of love and happiness regardless of what I was experiencing. This caused a state of empowerment and an emotional shift enabling me to enjoy and love everything I do, which then attracted to me what I love to do.

5. Power up your passwords.

When I became aware of the power of words and affirmations in creating our reality, I played with changing all my passwords for my website sign in's to words that expressed what I wanted to power up in my reality. Such as, the time I was writing my first book, I changed my passwords to reflect that goal in an already affirmed way. The password I chose was "I am an author" as the book entered completion, I moved on to other intentions, and I subsequently changed my passwords so that they reflected the new intentions as if achieved.

Just having to type in our user-names and passwords often on a computer is a way that we connect with a thought and a repetitious thought becomes a belief and a belief affects our actions and how we behave.

So try a few goal orientated passwords if you use the computer on a daily basis. "Step into the life you want to live as if you have always been there." This is something I do often and leave in place for roughly ninety days, so that like an affirmation I have repeated it often enough for it to sink into the subconscious.

6. Spend time in nature.

There is much to be said about our environment and whether we are influenced by it. I have found that we are unconsciously affected by nature, until we move to awareness of our human energy-body, whereby we learn to consciously participate in energy fields. Being out in nature, amidst the energy of natural surroundings removes stress and harmonizes our energy to align with the vibrational energy of earth.

Earth and the elements of earth communicate through an action of unseen energy waves that can often be felt when you travel to a place other than the one in which you spend most time. We feel the intricate connection we have with the elements and energy of nature in moments such as, hiking in mountains, walking in the woods and frolicking on the beach. The natural constructs of the energy of the moving ocean and the soft sand and warming sun are often known to have an effect of relaxation by transmuting stress. The Gaia theory is a relatively new theory that shows the connection of human consciousness and planetary consciousness into one big field of consciousness that is interdependent on each other for evolution.

Getting out into nature is a benefit for those who have a higher vibration, as it acts to ground one into this reality, so that they can continue to participate in this reality as opposed to feeling too detached from it. Higher vibrations are energy of light and the tendency of a light being is to move more in spirit existence than in physical reality. So nature has a twofold effect, it transmutes non-serving energy of a low vibration and also grounds those who find it hard to relate to what is going on around them.

7. Find at minimum half an hour of quite higher-self communion time everyday

Meditation has in my opinion, been one of those beneficial activities so misunderstood by the western world. The stigma placed on what it is and how to do it right, causes some people to question their own ability to meditate. Meditation is simple, just be still and allow yourself to observe whatever comes through your Energy-Body, with enough stillness and inactivity you will shift to the space of your higher-self.

As we begin to meditate we will usually experience a great deal of mind activity, somewhat like an inner party with hundreds of people(thoughts) in attendance, but the more you practice stillness those people (thoughts) without the fuel of your attention, leave and go home. Thoughts need energy to grow, and attention to nurture them, without this they can stay in seed formation, like the flower-seed you buy in a packet it will always be a flower seed until you perform some action on it.

Meditation harmonizes our energy-body with the energy of potential, which is the form of energy before we fuel it. The energy of potential is the frequency of our higher-self, and the energy flow within all creation. Time spent in mediation trains our brain frequencies out of the hectic motion of Beta brainwaves and causes us to operate more throughout our lives from the states of Alpha and Theta.

Each brainwave serves a particular function but when you attain the state of Alpha as a predominant brainwave, through the act of mediation, you are more harmoniously aligned with a;

- Relaxed body and mind
- Higher alignment with creativity
- Easier emotional processing
- Problem dissolving or aligning with the solutions
- Being one with life or, in the flow effortlessly attaining or moving through life.
- Higher learning abilities
- Healthy immune functioning

- Positive moods

Alpha brainwaves cultivate an increased awareness of our-self, body and mind, where we then discover, embody and intimately live life from a spirit-guided state. We have the key to open the door for our own higher-self presence to flow into our world.

8. Practice selective interaction.

While shifting to a higher vibration and developing awareness of resurfacing dense energy from within, we can still our activity by being present in the moment, but not becoming reactive to what is going on. There is a difference between giving attention to something and observation: the first is a direct connection whereby you merge your energy field with that to which you are giving attention, while the second is a detached but aware state, one in which you can then decide whether to flow your life source energy into what you are observing.

Often, we waste our energy by engaging in the many dramas that appear in our reality. We then have very little left for the co-creating that we feel in our heart. We can practice selective interaction and put a stop to some of the energy draining activities that occur within our days.

Less interaction with energy resurfacing allows the energy to flow on its way; this is not to say ignore anything, but be aware of it and honor its flow.

For instance, if we come across someone who always seems to irritate us, then only we can change the dynamics of that interaction. In place of our judgment, we can choose to see the person as a child of God who is learning to connect with their higher-self. From this sight, we can make a choice to always interact with this person from a place of compassion, and harmoniously guide them toward seeing the beauty of life itself.

9. Look for the Divine in everything.

As you come into alignment with embodying more of the energy of the Creator you emulate that energy and find its presence powerfully flowing in your daily life. Just this one act of bringing our human energy-body vibrations into an alignment with all that is of a Divine frequency serves to transmute the content of our energy field that is of a low dense or material world vibration. We know that divine will, which is stronger than human will, prevails over all manifestation.

Contemplate the thoughts in your head and evaluate them for the utmost Divine content. What I mean is, "Would Divine Source say, 'I can't do a certain thing?'" Nothing is unattainable to an energetic frequency of pure potentiality. This frequency of potential can be seen everywhere in existence as everything in existence was sourced from a potential.

We all channel this energy, and we can all discern in any moment, a potential that can be fueled and acted on. We can see Divinity when we look at how anything actually came into being.

Often we hurry through our days on a sort of rigid schedule, and we fail to stop and notice that within everything the light of the Divine is visible. A simple smile, the scent of a rose, and the warming rays of a beautiful sun, are Divine light that we can all be grateful for. Our move to recognizing this divinity and our gratitude of it will make sure that we receive more of it. Thus all that obscures Divine light fades from our reality and we find we have without any effort, put our attention on beauty, harmony, light and joy, and served to transform the energy that blocks the light of a Divine creation.

10. Know and alter non-serving beliefs

Picking and choosing what we believe determines the physical reality in which we live. This, in itself, is an empowering action within a world that often sets us up to play victim. Because, by unearthing old, non-serving beliefs and developing new beliefs;

• We then get to choose our life;
• We can consciously align our lives with health;
• We are able to believe in ourselves as successful beings;
• We can engage with wisdom in harmonious relationships and encounter them daily;
• We can choose only those beliefs that serve our attaining a passionate, joyful existence, and,
• We are able to lighten the load of energy density that we feel within our Energy-Body.

Unless we personally make those choices for ourselves, we will always be a victim to circumstances, situations and experiences that make us feel that they just happen to us, and not by us.

Chapter 10

Our Never-Ending Story to *Raise Our Vibration*

We have covered many topics in this book, about health and our own energy-body with regards to health.

We have looked at a number of energy healing modalities, some of which you may have already tried and others that you may now want to experience.

We have discovered that the government involvement in complementary and alternative medicine, is a positive and collective force for change that will benefit future generations.

We are now more aware that ingestion of GMO hidden in the structure of our food are something that we do have control over because we ultimately shop for the food that we eat.

We know that our vibration of health is something that is entirely ours to change and that we can or not, as is our choice, involve others in our matrix. But in essence, health is an ever-expanding state of growth both of a personal and a collective nature. Our own energy matrix is part of a bigger matrix of humanity.

As we individually and collectively raise our energy-body vibration we will individually and collectively experience the resulting realities of that new vibration.

We may stay at a new vibration for a short time or quickly move through to the next, if we experience no challenges or blocks to prevent us from doing so. We do not have to actually watch vibrations per-say but we can know our self well enough to notice any vibrational shifts as they occur in either an elevating or demoting way.

When we ascertain that something is not compatible with our higher vibration then we have the option to make another choice. This other choice is what leads to assimilating a new vibration.

The very idea that we can experience an energy blockage within our energy field, arises because we have a specific vision of who we are and know that we have yet to see its reflection. Any belief that we are experiencing an energy block will lead to an empowered place of being able to shift energy until we see more of own specific desired vision reflected.

Often a block occurs because we hold an outdated belief one that may have once served us, but at this present time it no longer does. These once serving beliefs cause boundaries that do not allow the idea of our-self as a higher-vibrating being to be fully expressed throughout our day.

We all experience this, as we continually project *our* concept of life, out to life itself. When I decide that beef is not healthy for my body, I have at some level chosen to do so, since another person may have none of the symptoms that I do.

Within my experience of life, and at this particular time in my life it serves me to experience that beef is not something I want to eat. Can I honestly say that I know why? "No I cannot." But I do feel that my awareness in experiencing these things and expressing my experience through the written word connects as inspiration with others having similar experiences. There will be people who relate at an inner core level with what I write, because an energy matrix is not a singular energy field but a connective web of energetic presences that experience life along the same lines. But in saying that, I am not advocating for others to adjust their presence and expression because of what I write but to find a kindred spirit who expresses and desires to honor authenticity for everyone on the matrix.

When we think of higher vibrational health we have to truly do what works for us. We know that within us are the best answers for any moment that we live. But, when we do not go within to listen to those answers, then we get those answers from our external reality. This information we receive from external sources, can be far different from what our higher-self guides us toward.

As I wrote in *Higher Vibrational Spirituality* many of us still live life, thinking we are the mind and that *mind* is the lead of our life. In reality we are not the mind, it is only the receiver of transferred information from our higher-self. Our higher-self is the energetic spirit essence of who we are and is of a higher vibration then who we are in physical form. This higher-self always communicates with its counterpart in physical reality but we are not always listening.

This is why learning how to hear this guidance from spirit provides a lifestyle, that offers direction of the best kind for our everyday life.

We actually get all of our ideas from our higher-self unless we are listening to other peoples ideas and continue to use them as guidance.

When we understand how we actually exist on physical and spiritual levels and how they tie together, we are in a better state to allow the higher vibrations of our higher-self to guide our journey.

When we look at our present state of health and then recall a time in which we were healthier, because of the perceived ability to know that everything simultaneously exists; both the healthy and the now less healthy state, can both still be seen to exist. I say *perceived ability to exist*, because as of yet not too many people grasp this.

When we honor the perception that we are healthy on some level of existence and it is still available to us, even if we do not feel or see that physically now, we can also perceive that we are in a place between the spectrum of *healthy me* and *unhealthy me* now. If we wish to expand the *me* into the healthy state that still exists then we can focus and set our intention toward that healthy state.

It then becomes a matter of trust and surrender that the higher-self recognizes the want, and knows the passion within our intention for health and so it will be.

It is then that we allow the higher self to do its work. Its work to deliver to us our vibration of health. We do not need to know how this will occur or when this will occur because the very fact that we are the human aspect of this spiritual/physical experience, shows it is not our place to direct but it is our place to receive the help of our higher-self on our journey.

If you intend for a healthy state and want to be the director of creating that healthy state, by demanding and stating how it should occur, you will miss the inflowing communication of higher-self guiding you to your healthy state.

We know that we are all ever-expanding and growing as we experience and continue our work at the leading edge of human existence. The uncharted territories that humans get into, are those that have already been experienced by civilizations before us. They are those that are presently experienced by civilizations that we have yet to communicate with. We can intuit their simultaneous existence or simply believe they exist. In either case we walk the path of this experience as one human family, continuously honoring the path of our brother as a very real and valid experience that ultimately helps us all.

There will always be choices that we have to make, situations to work through and discoveries that will unfold. Life itself will not bore us and yet in any given moment we may choose boredom. Life is not out to harm us and yet in any given moment we may feel harmed.

When we are aware of our choices within any given moment then we step into an empowered place of consciously making choices. What-ever choice we make it alters who we are and we become the new *us* from that point forward.

Essentially, we continuously transform because of every choice we make or even decide not to make!. As we begin to see this process within how we actually experience life, we are then empowered to see how everyday life is no more than a construct of our perception and that, because of its fluid state, life is anything that we intently focus on.

Real becomes illusion and illusion becomes real, because of this we move beyond the confines of only a physical existence and embody the energy of our higher-self,. Now we see the sights the higher-self sees, we know the way the higher-self knows and we exist in dimensions that the higher-self exists.

Because healing is wholeness, meaning unification of mind, body and spirit in a harmony, we live a never-ending story of raising our vibration. We live continually in a flux of healing and experience, healing and experience.

Healing is our way of ascension to the highest vibration that we can embody within physical form, We are not *aiming* to embody this spiritual vibration but consciously practicing surrender to do so. Surrender of our egoistic control of the very life we live.

The never-ending story as I see it.

We are all eminent sparks send forth from the one God source. This source I like to call, the Frequency of the Creator. Our inner essence is always unified with the

Frequency of the Creator and cherished as being a very real and valid presence within the whole.

Because the energy of the Creator is for creation, we too at the inner depths of our being carry that creative spirit frequency. Our journey to earth was not for the heck of it but so that the Creator could expand the vibration of love and grow in presence.

During that expansion we agreed to populate a place called earth which existed at a denser vibration than the one that we held. In order to populate earth we agreed to travel through the veil to a denser vibration while remaining by way of vibrational dimensions connected to our source the Creator from whence we came.

This eternal connection meant we could learn to shine what light we could from us and learn to bring in more of this vibrational light so that this small planet in the universe would one day shine like a brilliant star.

A journey of descent of our higher-vibrational state into a dimension, of denser vibrations. Here we would arrive in a forgetful state and school our-self, through the energy vibrations of hate, jealousy, judgment, fear, etc. We would experiment with emotions and thoughts and live in a state of physical formation that often times gave us that feeling of not being home. This was because our true inner nature was and is, as a free spirit, without the boundaries, that being a human has.

Would we succumb to the denser vibration of earth and live eternally cut off from the source of life and truly live in hell were there is no growth, expansion or moment beyond the one we hold? Or would we learn the lessons necessary for a complete embodiment of The Frequency of God and watch as the earth transformed into heaven before our eyes.

The ever pulsing light/energy of the Creator has never given up on the God sparks who live that journey.

We are at the dawn of realizing that we are a God spark and that we do have the power of creative ability beyond the limits of these dimensional frequencies that surround earth. Because of that we are shifting our vibration, both individually and collectively, so that the next level of creation or a higher dimension is born before our very eyes.

For many of us, we have released the hold of this third dimension and it's trappings of material and egoistic gains. We have held on to that tiny spark within and vowed to expand its presence here, where it belongs.

We see that life here, even with free-will choices can bring about more of the same because people have come to enjoy the role of controller over others and this breeds more people who play the role of victim.

We will remain separated from our inner higher-self while wearing the role of victim because our higher-self is powerful and not aligned with this role we play.

There are many scenarios and experiences in which this journey allows us to take part. In some we easily see the lesson learned by our participation and in others the lesson is more elusive. But when we look at the situations and experiences as a path toward a higher vibration we are then able to discern whether to continue or change course.

We now have many enlightening stories, of masters who have come to show us how to unify with our higher-self. And still many people have yet to grasp that they have the awesome power of the Creator at the core of their being.

But on the same hand there are people who have realized the presence of their lighter higher-self and they cultivate its expression in everyday that they live. This higher vibration ushers in to all of humanity, that we are on a single unified journey and that what occurs for one affects all of us.

We can see our life here on this planet from the view of our higher-self and as we continually express this view it alters the collective view of humanity.

We cannot fully bring through the full essence of the Divine until we release the energetic hold that the denser vibrations have on us.

The way we do this is through honoring experiences that we have in our everyday life, and using them to chose the Divine way.

Each experience, encounter and relationship is a lesson to help us shift from within our energy field, a vibration that causes repetition of circumstances which lack Divine light. In shifting the energy blocks within our field we embody more of the light of our higher-self.

We are not being punished by our journey here but are experiencing the full expression of God in many forms.

We have essentially come here to heal the divide living life on earth causes with the vibrations of our inner higher-self.

This healing is an inner healing which removes all that causes our perception to see us as separate. We heal every separatist thought, idea and action. We heal every emotion that causes us to feel separate from our God self. We heal our heart center from its pain. We heal the mind from cultivating thoughts and beliefs that are alternative to who we are at our core. We heal the body of sickness and disease; the signs that our energy vibrations are not bringing in, the light of the Divine.

Healing occurs when we ask, when we ask of our higher-self and when we listen to that inner guidance from spirit.

We will never find the answer to our spiritual expansion in the material gains we make, the dramas that we get sucked into, or the ego's quest to keep us blinded to the light. Were we place our attention, is key to what expands in our life.

Many of us have forgotten that we have our own guidance system within and we started to equate how much money we have, and the sense of fulfillment that money brings, with the only true source of spiritual nourishment and love. And yet, our gift of free-will, will never be taken from us. We can continue to find illusory states, to give us momentary satisfaction or we can choose to live authentically as the Divine essence that we really are.

When we go beyond the considered norm of a mass state of consciousness and take personal responsibility for everything that has occurred and is yet to occur in our life. Only then, will we step into alignment with receiving guidance from our God self.

We are here to honor the journey of spirit. The journey to move in uncharted ways and to not be stuck in the story but to write the healing that will bring us all back to an empowered state of existence.

Every thought travels as energy to imprint the field of our conscious existence. Every belief serves up itself. Every fear will come into being because we enact the vibration of it doing so. Every disease takes hold because we strengthen the pattern of its existence.

Our personal part of the entire existence-experience, recognizes its-self in our everyday reflection, as co-creator of realities, this occurs until such time as the reflection merges with the reflected and we exist as All.

It is we who have forgotten where our power is and more importantly how to use it, but as we live and grow we return to that powerful state of existence, reaping the rewards of health in all areas of our life.

Acknowledgments

(http://getunstuck.university1000.com/self-improvement/what-is-your-vibrational-frequency)

www.chakrashack.com,

www.seqclinic.com

Dr. Frank Kinslow

Http://www.danuforest.co.uk

http://www.mexconnect.com

http://www.Health.harvard.edu

http://www.Yoga.about.com

http://www.slimhealthysexy.com

http://www.leg.state.vt.us/statutes/fullsection.cfm?Title=06&Chapter=035&Section=00641

https://www.leahy.senate.gov/issues/agriculture-nutrition-and-dairy

http://foodmatters.tv/articles-1/10-amazing-health-benefits-of-bee-pollen